Applying Comparative Effectiveness Data to Medical Decision Making

Carl V. Asche

Editor

Applying Comparative Effectiveness Data to Medical Decision Making

A Practical Guide

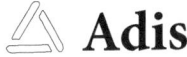 Adis

Editor
Carl V. Asche
Research Professor, Director of Center for Outcomes Research
Department of Pharmacy Systems, Outcomes and Policy
Affiliate Faculty, Center for Pharmacoepidemiology
and Pharmacoeconomic Research, University of Illinois
at Chicago College of Pharmacy
Chicago, IL
USA

Research Affiliate
Centre on Aging, University of Victoria
Victoria
British Columbia

ISBN 978-3-319-22064-2   ISBN 978-3-319-23329-1   (eBook)
DOI 10.1007/978-3-319-23329-1

Library of Congress Control Number: 2015956409

Springer Cham Heidelberg New York Dordrecht London

Printed on acid-free paper

Adis is a brand of Springer

Springer International Publishing AG Switzerland is part of Springer Science+Business Media
(www.springer.com)

Contents

Contributors

Carl V. Asche, PhD Research Professor, Director of Center for Outcomes Research, Department of Pharmacy Systems, Outcomes and Policy, Affiliate Faculty, Center for Pharmacoepidemiology and Pharmacoeconomic Research, University of Illinois at Chicago College of Pharmacy, Chicago, IL, USA

Research Affiliate, Centre on Aging, University of Victoria, Victoria, British Columbia

Jaeyong Bae, PhD Public Health and Health Education Programs, School of Nursing and Health Studies, Northern Illinois University, DeKalb, IL, USA

Andy Bland, MD HSHS Medical Group, Springfield, IL, USA

Department of Internal Medicine, University of Illinois College of Medicine at Peoria, Peoria, IL, USA

Hospital & Health Care, Springfield, IL, USA

James F. Graumlich, MD Department of Internal Medicine, University of Illinois College of Medicine at Peoria, Peoria, IL, USA

Jessica Hanks, MD Department of Internal Medicine and Pediatrics, University of Illinois College of Medicine at Peoria, Peoria, IL, USA

Nikhil R. Kalva, MD Department of Internal Medicine, University of Illinois College of Medicine at Peoria, Peoria, IL, USA

Inkyu K. Kim, PhD Battelle Memorial Institute, Atlanta, GA, USA

Minchul Kim, PhD Center for Outcomes Research, Department of Internal Medicine, University of Illinois College of Medicine at Peoria, Peoria, IL, USA

Carmen S. Kirkness, PhD Center for Outcomes Research, Department of Internal Medicine, University of Illinois College of Medicine at Peoria, Peoria, IL, USA

Matt Mischler, MD Department of Internal Medicine and Pediatrics, University of Illinois College of Medicine at Peoria, Peoria, IL, USA

Bonnie Paris, PhD Center for Outcomes Research, Department of Internal Medicine, University of Illinois College of Medicine at Peoria, Peoria, IL, USA

Jinma Ren, PhD Center for Outcomes Research, Department of Internal Medicine, University of Illinois College of Medicine at Peoria, Peoria, IL, USA

Chapter 1
Introduction to Comparative Effectiveness Research

Carmen S. Kirkness

Abstract Health expenditures in the United States have increased without the equal improvement in quality. Comparative effectiveness research (CER), the evaluation of health-care outcomes that are achieved relative to the cost incurred, is seen as an approach that would help stem the ever-increasing health-care costs. The CER initiative has been denoted as a novel way to improve health-care decisions made by patients, physicians, and other stakeholders. Large efforts have been and continue to be made to establish this initiative. These efforts were formalized by financial support confirmed through the American Recovery and Reinvestment Act (2009) and the establishment of a Patient-Centered Outcomes Research Institute (PCORI) to support CER through evidence generation. This chapter will serve to introduce CER definitions, terminology, role, characteristics, and the level of evidence specific to CER, to individuals

Past Health-Care Costs

Increasing costs and system inefficiencies in the United States have led to the pursuit of improved quality of care and the evaluation of the relative value of medical treatments [1]. In the past decade, the total health expenditure has doubled, reaching $2.7 trillion ($8,680 per person), which represented 17.9 % of the nation's gross domestic product (GDP) in 2011 [2]. Despite the increase of funds, the United States underperforms other advanced nations on important health measures. This has led to a national focus on improving the quality of care while decreasing the cost.

Several seminal events have detailed a national research initiative to support better decision making about interventions by physicians and patients in health care [3]. The American Recovery and Reinvestment Act (ARRA) of 2009 formalized this initiative by allotting $1.1 billion toward this research initiative, which

C.S. Kirkness, PhD
Center for Outcomes Research, Department of Medicine,
University of Illinois College of Medicine at Peoria, Peoria, IL, USA
e-mail: csk@uic.edu

© Springer International Publishing Switzerland 2016   1
C. Asche (ed.), *Applying Comparative Effectiveness Data to Medical
Decision Making: A Practical Guide*, DOI 10.1007/978-3-319-23329-1_1

became known as comparative effectiveness research (CER). "The law states that the funding will be used for the conduct, support, or synthesis of research that compares the clinical outcomes, effectiveness, and appropriateness of items, services, and procedures used to prevent, diagnose, or treat diseases, disorders, and other health conditions and for encouraging the development and use of clinical registries, clinical data networks, and other forms of electronic health data that can be used to generate or obtain outcomes data" [4]. CER initiative is significant because it is a high-profile national research commitment to promote and improve decision making by patients and their physicians [5]. The CER initiative has now expanded to organizations beyond the government and includes medical associations, the health industry, health plan providers, and purchasers, to name a few. As a broad-based initiative, the CER hopes to mobilize system change by improving the effectiveness of care and suspending the growth in health-care costs by providing applicable real-world information for improved decision making [5]. Solidifying this initiative was the establishment of an independent institute to conduct comparative effectiveness research (CER), the Patient-Centered Outcomes Research Institute (PCORI), in March of 2010. This institute is a nonprofit corporation that is administered through a 19-member board of governors that includes the directors of the National Institutes of Health (NIH) and the Agency for Healthcare Research and Quality (AHRQ), patient representatives, physicians, private payers, medical industry representatives, health researchers, federal government representatives, and a 17-member "Methodology Committee" that includes scientific experts in clinical research, biostatistics, genomics, and research methodologies [6].

Efficacy Versus Effectiveness

The evaluation of medical interventions is critical to provide evidence of the benefits and harms of the interventions. The conditions under which the medical intervention is evaluated determine how generalizable that study can be when applied to current practice. They range from studies that have extremely controlled and restrictive conditions (efficacy studies) to those that evaluate an intervention in the real-world circumstances under which people actually use it (effectiveness studies). Historically, the effects of medical interventions on health have been evaluated based on efficacy. Efficacy studies determine whether an intervention produces the expected result under restrictive and controlled conditions in order to maximize the likelihood that the true effect will be evident if it indeed exists [7]. Effectiveness studies are at the other end of the continuum and are the evaluation of treatments in practice. The benefit of effectiveness studies is that the results can be applied to a broader population than efficacy studies, and thus these studies provide evidence that has great utility in health-care decisions for multiple stakeholders (providers, patients, and health care insurance providers).

Defining Comparative Effectiveness Research

The simple definition of CER is the comparison of two or more different health-care interventions' effectiveness within a defined set of individuals in real-world clinical settings. Organization-specific definitions of CER shown in Table 1.1 provide comprehensive definitions to outline the characteristics of the research that included the organization's CER. These definitions inform the public of the focus of their research and its importance in their lives. The definitions for various organizations share similarities and differences.

Table 1.1 Organization specific definitions of CER

Organization	Definition
Institute of Medicine [8] (IOM)	CER is the generation and synthesis of evidence that compares the benefits and harms of alternative methods to prevent, diagnose, treat and monitor a clinical condition, or to improve the delivery of care. The purpose of CER is to assist consumers, clinicians, purchasers, and policy makers to make informed decisions that will improve health care at both the individual and population levels
AHRQ [7]	Comparative effectiveness research is designed to inform health-care decisions by providing evidence on the effectiveness, benefits, and harms of different treatment options. The evidence is generated from research studies that compare drugs, medical devices, tests, surgeries, or ways to deliver health care
NIH [9]	Comparative effectiveness research is the conduct and synthesis of systematic research comparing different interventions and strategies to prevent, diagnose, treat and monitor health conditions. The purpose of this research is to inform patients, providers, and decision makers, responding to their expressed needs, about which interventions are most effective for which patients under specific circumstances. To provide this information, comparative effectiveness research must assess a comprehensive array of health-related outcomes for diverse patient populations
Federal Coordinating Council for Comparative Effectiveness Research [10, 11]	The Federal Coordinating Council for Comparative Effectiveness Research defines CER as "the conduct and synthesis of research comparing the benefits and harms of different interventions and strategies to prevent, diagnose, treat and monitor health conditions in 'real world' settings." The interventions and strategies studied range from medicine and device comparisons to diagnostic testing, behavioral change, and delivery system strategy analyses"
PCORI [6]	Although there are prioritized research areas, broadly CER includes research on various disease conditions (rare and not rare), health technologies, and the continuum of health-care services, settings, and deliveries

Role of Comparative Effectiveness Research

The role of CER is to inform decision making using a range of research tools and methods. As defined by the Institute of Medicine (IOM), it is to "assist consumers, clinicians, purchasers, and policymakers to make informed decisions that will improve healthcare at both the individual and population levels" [5]. These include systematic reviews of existing studies and evidence, modeling to simulate effects of interventions on different populations, head-to-head clinical trials comparing one treatment to another, and studies using data available from registries, electronic health records, administrative records, and other databases.

Although a broad scope of research defines comparative effective research, the central tenet of CER is to determine which treatment works, for whom, and under what conditions it works best. The following six characteristics, developed by the IOM, describe the elements that define a CER study. At least one characteristic should be present for a study to be considered CER [8].

The six characteristics of CER as defined by the IOM [8]:

1. CER directly informs a specific clinical decision (patient perspective) or a health policy decision (population perspective).
2. CER results are described at the population and subgroup levels.
3. CER compares at least two alternative interventions, each with the potential to be "best practice."
4. CER employs methods and data sources appropriate for the decision of interest.
5. CER is conducted in settings that are similar to those in which the intervention will be used in practice.
6. CER measures outcomes—both benefits and harms—that are important to patients.

CER directly informs a specific clinical decision (patient perspective) or a health policy decision (population perspective)

Questions that evaluate the health and health care of an individual patient or a population are important components that fulfill the goal of CER to identify what works best and for whom. The scopes of the studies include preventive, screening, diagnostic, therapeutic, monitoring, rehabilitative intervention, or policy-focused studies that synthesize knowledge or evaluate public health programs or initiatives involving the organization, delivery, or payment for health services.

CER results are described at the population and subgroup levels.

The evaluation of subgroups and the use of clinical prediction rules to identify patients who are likely to benefit from an intervention are important for the application of CER results to individual patients. These evaluations are intended to aid health decisions being made by providers and patients in the determination of whether the treatment can be individualized to the intended patient. In areas of health care that are rapidly developing, such as genomics and other biomedical sciences, the opportunity to develop individual targeted therapies and expand the application of personalized medicine is the greatest. Focusing on interventions that target individual patient decisions is a process that diverges greatly from decisions based on the results of clinical trials, where the results are expressed as the average group effect and are difficult to translate to individuals.

CER compares at least two alternative interventions, each with the potential to be "best practice."

Translating evidence to individual patients requires intervention comparisons that patients and providers can apply to their cases. Prior to CER, the accepted standard for clinical decisions was randomized controlled trial (RCT) studies that compared an intervention to a placebo and used a very restricted and homogeneous population. This type of study demonstrates whether the intervention is safe and efficacious and establishes "does it work?" CER studies seek to expand the comparison to establish whether one intervention is better than the other and for whom it works better. To make these conclusions, CER studies compare a test intervention with a viable alternative in subgroups of people that may not have been included in the RCT. Accepted viable CER comparators could be different intervention modes (surgery versus drug) or the evaluation of an intervention in the current standards of clinical practice.

CER comparisons can also extend to the evaluation of the clinical and resource effects of health-care delivery. Comparators that may be used in these situations may be medical benefit designs, integrated organizational models, population health models, and cost-sharing techniques.

CER employs methods and data sources appropriate for the decision of interest.

Methods

The three primary research categories applicable to CER are experimental studies (randomized controlled trials), nonexperimental studies (nonrandomized and observational), and synthesis studies (systematic reviews and meta-analysis, technology assessments, and decision analysis). These categories will briefly be described here with further discussion.

Experimental research involves a treatment, procedure, or program that is intentionally introduced, and a result or outcome is observed. The randomized clinical trial (RCT) is a classic experimental study design to be used to determine whether a difference exists between two or more groups. This design is conducted within a setting that is controlled, to a certain extent, by enrolling patients who meet pre-specified criteria and provide informed consent. A defining characteristic of an RCT is the random allocation of participants to the experimental group or the comparison group. An example of an experimental study that constitutes a method of CER is a head-to-head trial. This RCT study compares two groups of people with the same disease; one group receives an active intervention, while the other group does not. Other CER study designs in this category are cluster randomized, adaptive designs, and pragmatic trials.

Nonexperimental research consists of studies that collect data by observation, without making changes or introducing treatments. Observational research includes prospective and retrospective cohort studies, case-control studies, and case series analyses. The advantages of observational studies are that the population being studied can be diverse, treatments are more likely to be delivered in a manner consistent with clinical practice, and treatments that may be unethical to withhold in an RCT study design can be investigated. This study type is more in line with the goals of CER; research conducted in a real-life situation is easier to extrapolate to a real-life patient problem. The disadvantage of observational studies occurs as a result of the lack of randomization: group differences are expected, introducing a risk that the difference in outcomes could be due to the initial differences between patient groups. Methodologies to minimize this disadvantage are progressing and have been propelled forward with the advancement of electronic data collection in registry and database studies.

Relevant evidence that informs real-world health care decisions for stakeholders is a central tenet of CER. The plethora of available evidence requires evidence synthesis in the form of systematic reviews, meta-analysis, technology assessments, and decision analysis studies. These studies summarize the information from more than one study and are required to have systematic review strategies that are transparent and consistent, which allows valid comparisons of effectiveness. In turn, this methodological rigor allows these documents to become primary sources of information for stakeholders to make confident decisions [9, 10].

Data Sources

CER data is derived from multiple different existing sources that are readily accessed as a result of computers and health information technology. This includes information from the patient interaction in the health system, administrative claims data from large national insurers, the patient's electronic medical record that contains the standard medical and clinical data gathered in one provider's office, and the electronic health record that is a comprehensive collection of all of a patient's medical records. Another source includes patient registries, a collection of information about individuals in a standardized way using observational research methods. Registries can be focused on a specific diagnosis or condition and are used to identify people who may be underrepresented in research studies and for tracking of outcomes from clinical practice interventions [11].

CER is conducted in settings that are similar to those in which the intervention will be used in practice.

"Consistent with the definition of effectiveness, the settings of CER studies are a defining characteristic [8]." Studying interventions in a setting that reflects the current practice setting has the benefit of translating and disseminating CER findings in a timely and interpretable manner.

CER measures outcomes—both benefits and harms—that are important to patients.

The involvement of the patient is a priority for CER. The value of CER is in influencing real-world decision making. Therefore, determination of the net benefit (benefit-harm ratio) of the intervention is vital. The net-benefit ratio is inclusive of the harms or risks associated with the outcome of interest, and it is often measured by patient-reported outcomes (a patient's perception of an outcome). Patient-reported outcomes are necessary in the net-benefit evaluation because these outcomes often differ from clinical outcomes.

Patient Involvement

A defining feature of CER is the patient involvement that is a critical distinction from the traditional models of health research. In the traditional model, research questions are developed by scientists and experts and based on their opinions; they determine what outcomes and interventions are important for the patient. In this model, patients are passive participants in the research process, and this has resulted in research findings that are poorly aligned with the information important to patients. The role of the patient is instrumental to CER; therefore, research is that relevant and communicable to the patient, the caregiver, and the consumer is required. From the beginning of the research process, the conceptualization of the research question, patient beliefs are incorporated into CER through the active involvement of consumers, patients, and caregivers. Patient involvement is needed throughout the research project, ending with the implementation and the dissemination of findings.

The term "stakeholder" is broadly used in CER to define "individuals, organizations or communities that have a direct interest in the process and outcome of a project, research or policy endeavor" [12]. Stakeholders may be patients, their caregivers, health-care providers and delivery systems, patient advocates, policy makers, and consumers. Stakeholders frequently have limited experience in research. Engaging stakeholders in the research process requires education, training, and support. Table 1.2 outlines several programs that have been developed to help prepare stakeholders for their role in research.

Level of Evidence for CER

The nature of CER research requires study methodologies that address large and broad populations of patients in a usual-care setting while also being time sensitive so that decisions based on the results are being made with the most current available evidence. The assessment of the strength of the body of evidence is directly related to the confidence in the decision that can be made. The use of systematic grading criteria provides an accepted standard of evaluation by which to draw conclusions and transparently report the findings. Historically, levels of evidence have used a hierarchical study design model that places randomized controlled trials and meta-analysis at the top of the model. In CER studies, a more comprehensive evaluation of the evidence is recommended for decision makers.

The Evidence-based Practice Center (EPC) Program that is supported by the Agency for Healthcare Research and Quality (AHRQ) is responsible for developing

Table 1.2 Programs that have been developed to help prepare stakeholders for their role in research

Program	Function	Website
US Cochrane Center, Consumers United for Evidence-based Healthcare	A web-based course to help consumers understand the fundamentals of evidence-based health care	https://us.cochrane.org/ understanding-evidence-based-healthcare-foundation-action
National Breast Cancer Coalition's Project LEAD Institute	A science education program for breast cancer advocates and Quality Care Project LEAD	http://www.breastcancerdeadline2020.org/ get-involved/training/project-lead/ project-lead-institute.html
DOD Breast Cancer Research Program's peer review process	A web-based site to involve consumer advocates	http://cdmrp.army.mil/cwg/default.shtml
FDA's Patient Network	FDA staff offers training and support to patient representatives about policies, procedures, and regulations	http://www.fda.gov/ForPatients/About/ ucm412709.htm
Stakeholder Guide 2014	Guide to encourage patients, researchers, clinicians, and others to become involved in its Effective Health Care (EHC) Program	www.effectivehealthcare.ahrq.gov

and updating recommended guidelines for level of evidence assessment in CER studies. The EPC method is one system for reporting results and grading the related strength of evidence, and it presents a consistent, transparent process to document and report the most important summary information about a body of literature. The *EPC Methods Guide for Effectiveness and Comparative Effectiveness Reviews* (2014) provides detailed guidance on the systematic review of drugs, devices, and other preventive and therapeutic interventions [10]. The current recommendations will be briefly discussed, but due to the rapid evolution of CER methodologies, future updates to these recommendations are expected.

The EPC's method recommends multiple-component criteria for establishing the strength of evidence (SOE) in CER studies. The EPC method is largely based on the GRADE (Grading of Recommendations Assessment, Development and Evaluation) system [12] that has been widely adopted as an approach to rating confidence in estimates of effect the quality of evidence and guidance for practice. In the EPC method, there are five main specific domains, including study limitations, directness, consistency, precision, and reporting bias as described by domain and definition from the *Methods Guide for Effectiveness and Comparative Effectiveness Reviews* [12] shown in Table 1.3.

Table 1.3 Domains and definitions for strength of evidence rating

Domain	Definition

Study limitations	Study limitations is the degree to which the included studies for a given outcome have a high likelihood of adequate protection against bias (i.e., good internal validity), assessed through two main elements:
	    Study design: Whether RCTs or other designs such as nonexperimental or observational studies
	    Study conduct: Aggregation of ratings of risk of bias of the individual

Directness	Directness relates to (a) whether evidence links interventions directly to a health outcome of specific importance for the review and (b) for comparative studies, whether the comparisons are based on head-to-head studies Indirectness always implies that more than one body of evidence is required to link interventions to the most important health outcome

Consistency	Consistency is the degree to which studies find either the same direction or similar magnitude of effect. EPCs can assess this through two main elements:
	    Direction of effect: Effect sizes have the same sign (i.e., are on the same side of no effect or a minimally important difference [MID])
	    Magnitude of effect: The range of effect sizes is similar. EPCs may consider the overlap of confidence intervals (CIs) when making this evaluation
	The importance of direction vs. magnitude of effect will depend on the key question and EPC judgments

Precision	Precision is the degree of certainty surrounding an effect estimate with respect to a given outcome, based on the sufficiency of sample size and number of events:
	    A body of evidence will generally be imprecise if the optimal information size (OIS) is not met. OIS refers to the minimum number of patients (and events when assessing dichotomous outcomes) needed for an evidence base to be considered adequately powered
	    If EPCs performed a meta-analysis, then EPCs may also consider whether the CI crossed a threshold for an MID
	    If a meta-analysis is infeasible or inappropriate, EPCs may consider the narrowness of the range of CIs or the significance level of p-values in the individual studies in the evidence base

Reporting bias	Reporting bias results from selectively publishing or reporting research findings based on the favorability of direction or magnitude of effect. It includes:
	    Study publication bias, i.e., nonreporting of the full study
	    Selective outcome reporting bias, i.e., nonreporting (or incomplete reporting) of planned outcomes or reporting of unplanned outcomes
	    Selective analysis reporting bias, i.e., reporting of one or more favorable analyses for a given outcome while not reporting other, less favorable analyses
	Assessment of reporting bias for individual studies depends on many factors, e.g., availability of study protocols, unpublished study documents, and patient-level data. Detecting such bias is likely with access to all relevant documentation and data pertaining to a journal publication, but such access is rarely available
	Because methods to detect reporting bias in observational studies are less certain, this guidance does not require EPCs to assess it for such studies

EPC Evidence-based Practice Center
Definitions are direct quotations from: Ref. [10]. Chapter 15, pages 320–321. Available at: www.effectivehealthcare.ahrq.gov

Table 1.4 Strength of evidence grades and definitions

Grade	Definition
High	We are confident that the estimate of effect lies close to the true effect for this outcome The body of evidence has few or no deficiencies. We believe that the findings are stable, i.e., another study would not change the conclusions
Moderate	We are moderately confident that the estimate of effect lies close to the true effect for this outcome The body of evidence has some deficiencies. We believe that the findings are likely to be stable, but some doubt remains
Low	We have limited confidence that the estimate of effect lies close to the true effect for this outcome The body of evidence has major or numerous deficiencies (or both). We believe that additional evidence is needed before concluding either that the findings are stable or that the estimate of effect is close to the true effect
Insufficient	We have no evidence, we are unable to estimate an effect, or we have no confidence in the estimate of effect for this outcome. No evidence is available or the body of evidence has unacceptable deficiencies, precluding reaching a conclusion

Strength of Evidence Grades

EPCs assess individual domain scores and establish overall strength of evidence grades relevant to each key question. The overall grade for the strength of evidence is a global assessment that includes a judgment about the strength of the evidence for each major benefit and harm that is relevant to stakeholders in the setting in which the recommendations are being made [13]. The EPC method of strength of evidence consists of four grades: high, moderate, low, or insufficient. Each strength of evidence definition provided by the *Methods Guide for Effectiveness and Comparative Effectiveness Reviews* [10] is briefly described in Table 1.4. Two criteria, representing different conceptual frameworks, are required at each level. The first criterion determines the evaluator's judgment that the evidence reflects the true effect. The continuum of choices range from high to insufficient, with a high grade representing a clear, true effect level and with an insufficient grade stating that evaluators were unable reach a conclusion. The second criterion is "a subjective assessment of the likelihood that future research might affect the level of confidence in the estimate or actually change that estimate." It is also denoted by high, moderate, low, and insufficient grades [10, 13].

References

1. Keehan SP, Sisko AM, Truffer CJ et al (2011) National health spending projections through 2020: economic recovery and reform drive faster spending growth. Health Aff (Millwood) 30:1594–1605
2. Health, United States, 2013: with special feature on prescription drugs (2014) At http://www.cdc.gov/nchs/data/hus/hus13.pdf#112

3. Eden J, Wheatley B, McNeil B, Sox H (2008) Knowing what works in health care: a roadmap for the nation. National Academies Press, Washington, DC
4. The American Recovery and Reinvestment Act of 2009. The American Recovery and Reinvestment Act of 2009. At http://www.gpo.gov/fdsys/pkg/BILLS-111hr1enr/pdf/BILLS-111hr1enr.pdf. Accessed 12 Oct 2015
5. Sox HC, Greenfield S (2009) Comparative effectiveness research: a report from the Institute of Medicine. Ann Intern Med 151:203–205
6. Patient-centered outcome research institute: national priorities for research and research agenda (2012) At http://www.pcori.org/content/national-priorities-and-research-agenda. Accessed 14 Nov 2014
7. Velentgas P, Dreyer N, Nourjah P, Smith S, Torchia MM (2013) Developing a protocol for observational comparative effectiveness research: a User's guide. AfHRaQ, ed, Rockville
8. Medicine Io (2009) Initial national priorities for comparative effectiveness research Washington. National Academies Press, Washington, DC
9. Owens DK, Lohr KN, Atkins D, et al (2008) Grading the strength of a body of evidence when comparing medical interventions. In: Methods Guide for effectiveness and comparative effectiveness reviews. Rockville
10. Methods Guide for Effectiveness and Comparative Effectiveness Reviews [Internet] (2014) In: Quality, AfHRa, ed. Methods Guide for Effectiveness and Comparative Effectiveness Reviews. AHRQ Publication No. 10(14)-EHC063-EF. Agency for Healthcare Research and Quality, Rockville
11. NIH Clinical Reserch Trials and you (2014) List of registries. At http://www.nih.gov/health/clinicaltrials/registries.htm
12. Deverka PA, Lavallee DC, Desai PJ et al (2012) Stakeholder participation in comparative effectiveness research: defining a framework for effective engagement. J Comp Eff Res 1:181–194
13. Guyatt G, Oxman AD, Sultan S et al (2013) GRADE guidelines: 11. Making an overall rating of confidence in effect estimates for a single outcome and for all outcomes. J Clin Epidemiol 66:151–157

Chapter 2
Randomized Controlled Trials

Nikhil R. Kalva and James F. Graumlich

Abstract Comparative effectiveness research generates evidence from observational studies and randomized controlled trials. For many clinical questions, the observational study is an efficient design. Sometimes inherent biases in observational studies yield false results that require refutation by a randomized controlled trial. An illustrative example occurred with hormone replacement therapy in post-menopausal women. Numerous observational studies showed benefits of estrogen plus progesterone to prevent coronary heart disease and other adverse outcomes. A subsequent large, randomized controlled trial demonstrated that the harms of hormone replacement therapy exceeded the benefits. Randomized controlled trials play an important role in comparative effectiveness research. To understand this role, it is necessary to have knowledge about bias, ethics, efficacy, and effectiveness. The current chapter explains the benefits of randomization to reduce bias in the context of controlled clinical trials. There is also an explanation of the ethical principles that inform the design of trials. Finally, the chapter differentiates efficacy from effectiveness and explores trial design characteristics related to the differences.

Introduction

Comparative effectiveness evidence is generated from observational studies and randomized controlled trials. For many clinical questions, the observational study is an efficient design. Sometimes inherent biases in observational studies yield false results that require refutation by a randomized controlled trial. An illustrative example occurred with hormone replacement therapy in post-menopausal women. Numerous observational studies showed benefits of estrogen plus progesterone to prevent coronary heart disease and other adverse outcomes. A subsequent large, randomized controlled trial demonstrated that the harms of hormone replacement

N.R. Kalva, MD • J.F. Graumlich, MD (✉)
Department of Medicine, University of Illinois College of Medicine at Peoria, Peoria, IL, USA
e-mail: nkalva@uic.edu; jfg@uic.edu

© Springer International Publishing Switzerland 2016   13
C. Asche (ed.), *Applying Comparative Effectiveness Data to Medical
Decision Making: A Practical Guide*, DOI 10.1007/978-3-319-23329-1_2

therapy exceeded the benefits [19]. Randomized controlled trials play an important role in comparative effectiveness research. To understand this role, it is necessary to have knowledge about bias, ethics, efficacy, and effectiveness. The current chapter explains the benefits of randomization to reduce bias in the context of controlled clinical trials. There is also an explanation of the ethical principles that inform the design of trials. Finally, the chapter differentiates efficacy from effectiveness and explores trial design characteristics related to the differences.

What Is a Controlled Clinical Trial?

A clinical trial is an experiment on humans. The purpose of the experiment is to test the efficacy or effectiveness of an intervention. The broad definition of intervention includes drugs, therapeutic devices, or surgical procedures. In addition, interventions may include any health-care course of action under investigation, like education, behavior modification, prevention, diagnosis, or health-care delivery models. A controlled clinical trial has at least two interventions, called test treatment and control treatment. The participants who receive the test treatment are called the test group. The control group receives the control treatment. A diagram of a controlled clinical trial appears in Fig. 2.1. The design of the experiment is to compare the effects of test treatment with the effects of control treatment in comparable groups of humans. The effects of the interventions are quantified by the outcome measures. Examples of clinical trial outcomes appear in Table 2.1.

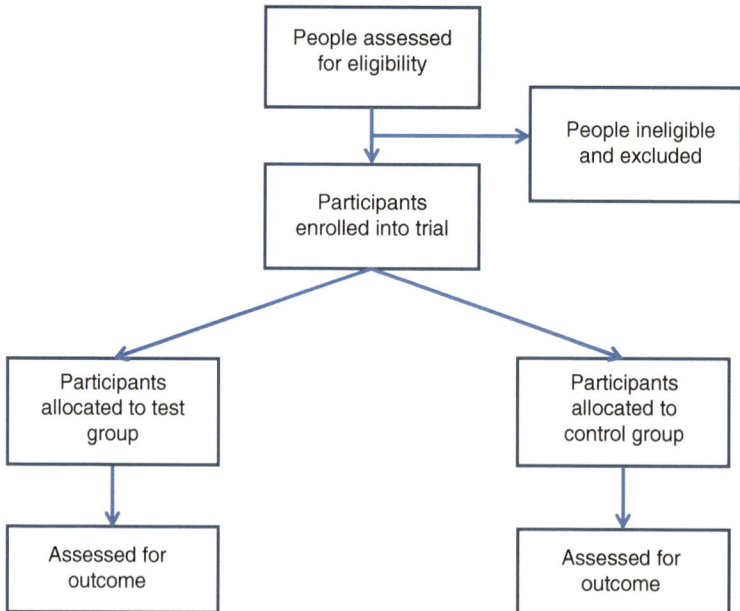

Fig. 2.1 Diagram of a controlled clinical trial

Table 2.1 Examples of outcomes (endpoints) used in clinical trials

Outcome (endpoint)	Type of variable	Effect size
Blood pressure Hemoglobin A1c	Continuous	Difference of means
All-cause mortality Acute myocardial infarction	Binary	Odds ratio, relative risk, or risk difference
Survival Progression-free survival	Time to occurrence	Kaplan-Meier statistic, Hazard ratio
Number of patients who leave a hospital against medical advice	Counts	Probability from Poisson or negative binomial model

Table 2.2 Examples of surrogate and clinical endpoints as outcome measures in clinical trials

Disease	Surrogate endpoint	Clinical endpoint
Cardiovascular	Blood pressure Cholesterol	Myocardial infarction, stroke, death
Diabetes mellitus	Hemoglobin A1c	Blindness from diabetic retinopathy, pain from diabetic neuropathy, amputation from diabetic peripheral vascular disease
Osteoporosis	Bone mineral density	Fractures
Glaucoma	Intraocular pressure	Blindness
Acquired Immunodeficiency Syndrome	CD4 count Viral load	Opportunistic infection, mortality
Cancer	Tumor volume	Mortality
Liver disease from acetaminophen intoxication	Acetaminophen concentration in blood	Liver transplant, death from liver failure

The outcomes of clinical trials may be further classified as biomarkers or endpoints. By definition, *a biomarker is a characteristic that is objectively measured and evaluated as an indicator of normal biological processes, pathogenic processes, or pharmacologic responses to a therapeutic intervention* [5]. A clinical endpoint is a characteristic or variable that reflects how a patient feels, functions, or survives [5]. In contrast to a clinically relevant endpoint, a surrogate endpoint is a biomarker that is intended to substitute for a clinical endpoint [5]. Table 2.2 shows examples of clinical endpoints and their corresponding surrogates.

The most important outcome measured in a clinical trial is called the primary endpoint. The investigator and statistician use the primary endpoint to estimate the sample size for the clinical trial. The sample size is the number of participants that need to be recruited and followed in the test group and the control group to have sufficient statistical power for tests of inference. Most clinical trials have one primary endpoint with multiple secondary endpoints. When there are additional primary endpoints, there is a loss of statistical power due to multiple comparisons. Trials with multiple primary endpoints usually require an increase in sample size in order to maintain statistical power.

Effect size is the measure of the difference in outcomes between the intervention groups. Commonly, effect size for a binary outcome is expressed as a statistic like relative risk, odds ratio, or risk difference. When the outcomes are continuous measures, then the statistic for effect size is the difference of means. When researchers measure time to occurrence of a binary outcome, then the relevant effect size may be a hazard ratio or Kaplan-Meier statistic. Examples of clinical trial outcomes and their related effect sizes appear in Table 2.1.

When a controlled clinical trial measures a difference in outcomes between the intervention groups, then there are three logical interpretations of the difference. The difference could be a true difference between the treatments or secondary to systematic error or chance variability. Systematic error, or bias, is a distortion of the estimated intervention effect size caused by inadequacies in the design, conduct, or analysis of a trial [6]. If the researcher minimizes bias and chance variability, then any difference in outcome measures is attributable to a true difference between test treatment and control.

One of the important causes of systematic error is selection bias. In observational studies of patients, the treatment selection is made by a clinician who seeks to optimize efficacy, maximize patient satisfaction, and minimize adverse effects and costs for individual patients. There is no attempt or desire to assign test treatment or control treatment to identical patients. As a consequence, the recipients of test or control treatment may differ in ways that are unrelated to treatment assignment. Selection bias occurs when prognostic factors related to treatment outcome are distributed unevenly between the test and control groups. The consequences of selection bias often are less favorable outcomes in the control group when compared to the test group. If an observational study measures a difference in outcomes between test and control groups, the researcher may not infer that the difference was due to treatment assignment because the difference may be attributable to bias.

Controlled clinical trials are also vulnerable to selection bias. An example of selection bias occurs in the following scenario. An investigator conducts a controlled clinical trial in patients with atrial fibrillation. The purpose of the trial is to compare new drug A versus control drug B for the prevention of stroke. If the investigator knows that the next patient enrolled in the trial will be assigned to drug B, then the investigator could knowingly or unconsciously offer drug B to older patients with higher risk for stroke. If this pattern of behavior persists, then the group of participants assigned to drug B would have a higher risk for stroke. At the end of the study, any reduction in strokes in the group assigned to drug A compared to drug B could be attributed to selection bias and not to a benefit of drug A.

What Is the Benefit of Randomization?

Random treatment assignment can overcome the problems of selection bias. When performed properly, random treatment assignment assures that the test and control treatment groups are identical for all measured and unmeasured participant characteristics and prognostic factors. Randomization is the process of assigning participants to treatment groups so that each participant has a known and usually an equal chance of being assigned to a given group. The intention of randomization is to ensure that the group assignment is unpredictable.

Randomization has two requirements: generation of an unpredictable allocation sequence and concealment of the allocation sequence from research personnel who enroll subjects. Sequentially enrolled participants are assigned to treatment groups in the order defined by the allocation sequence. The allocation sequence is unpredictable when it is random. Appropriate methods to generate a random allocation sequence use tables of random numbers or computer-generated random numbers. Examples of inappropriate allocation schemes include assignment to test treatment on even number days and control treatment on odd number days. Odd-even and other alternating assignment schemes do not avoid bias because they are highly predictable and subject to manipulation.

Meta-analyses have measured the benefit of randomization to the scientific validity of controlled clinical trials. When compared to randomized controlled trials with adequate generation of the random sequence, trials with inadequate generation have exaggerated and biased estimates of the effect size by 11 % [20].

The second requirement for randomization is allocation concealment. If the next assignment is known, then it is possible to delay or prevent enrollment of selected participants to ensure that they receive the treatment believed to be superior [11]. Allocation concealment means the participant and research personnel are unaware of the next assignment in the allocation sequence during the process of screening for eligibility and informed consent. The benefit of allocation concealment has been quantified. Randomized controlled trials with inadequate allocation concealment exaggerate the effect size by 7 % [20].

The main advantage of randomization is the elimination of selection bias. There are additional benefits to the validity of controlled clinical trials. Randomized allocation also facilitates blinding.

What Is the Benefit of Blinding?

Another cause of systematic error in clinical trials is ascertainment bias. The definition of ascertainment bias is *systematic distortion of the results of a randomized trial as a result of knowledge of the group assignment by the person assessing outcome, whether an investigator or the participant themselves* (http://www.consort-statement.org/resources/glossary). Preconceived positive or negative opinions about the intervention may influence how participants report the benefits or adverse effects of treatment. Likewise, research personnel are vulnerable to their preconceptions when assessing the outcomes of treatment. To avoid ascertainment bias, researchers use blinding, also called masking.

Double blind means the participants and the research personnel are unaware of the treatment allocation. The benefit of the double-blind design has been measured. When compared with trials with adequate double blind, trials without double blind exaggerate the effect size by 13 % [20].

What Are the Limitations of Randomized Controlled Trials?

Randomized controlled trials are advantageous to comparative effectiveness research because they measure effect size with minimal bias. The advantages must be considered in the context of limitations as well. Randomized controlled trials take a long time to start up and complete because of the necessary processes to enroll participants, follow them over time, and assess their outcomes [10]. For similar reasons, randomized controlled trials are expensive [8].

A case study will help to explain the advantages and limitations of randomized controlled trials for comparative effectiveness. ALLHAT (Antihypertensive and Lipid-Lowering treatment to prevent Heart Attack Trial) was a trial that had a profound influence on treatment guidelines for hypertension [3]. ALLHAT enrolled patients who were 55 years or older with hypertension plus other risk factors for coronary heart disease. The primary hypothesis of the antihypertensive trial was that the combined incidence of fatal coronary heart disease and nonfatal myocardial infarction would be lower in hypertensive patients randomized to amlodipine, lisinopril, or doxazosin than in those randomized to chlorthalidone. The statistical design accounted for three primary comparisons and required over 40,000 participants to achieve 82.5 % statistical power to test the primary hypothesis [7]. Because of the large sample size, ALLHAT required 623 clinical centers and 4 years to achieve the participant recruitment goal. After the end of recruitment, ALLHAT investigators followed participants for another 4 years before the results were analyzed and reported [1]. The size and duration of ALLHAT contributed to the cost of the trial. According to newspaper reports, the estimated cost of ALLHAT exceeded $100 million [12].

What Are the Ethical Considerations in the Design of Randomized Controlled Trials?

Randomized controlled trials are experiments on humans. Unfortunately, there is a history of disturbing incidents where investigators violated human rights. In response to violations, the National Commission for Protection of Human Subjects of Biomedical and Behavioral Research identified ethical principles to safeguard human research participants. The commission's report, published in 1979, is known as the Belmont Report [18].

The Belmont Report identified three ethical principles that govern the design and conduct of human research. The principles are justice, respect for persons, and beneficence. These three principles are the foundation for regulations that protect the rights of human research participants. In many countries, governmental regulations empower research ethics committees to approve and monitor clinical research. In the United States, research ethics committees are called institutional review boards [4]. The purpose of the institutional review board is to protect human research participants and assure investigator compliance with ethical principles.

The first principle, respect for persons, recognizes the rights of participants to be informed about their treatment options. The researcher must respect individual autonomy and the participant's right to self-determination. When applied to randomized controlled trials, the principle of respect for persons means the participant must give voluntary and informed consent. Participants have the corollary right to withdraw from the clinical trial at any time. One of the major duties of institutional review boards is to assure that researchers obtain and document informed consent from every research participant.

Justice is the second principle of ethics in clinical research. Under the principle of justice, the benefits and burdens of research must be distributed equally among equals. In the context of randomized controlled trials, justice applies to the selection of research participants.

Institutional review boards require researchers to enroll participants without coercion and to protect the rights of vulnerable individuals.

The third principle, beneficence, requires the researcher to do no harm. In clinical research, it is common to have incomplete foreknowledge of all potential harms or benefits of the test intervention. Oftentimes, the aims of clinical research are to quantify the probability of benefit and the risk of harm. The principle of beneficence requires the researcher to maximize possible benefits and minimize possible harms. Clinical trial protocols must include methods to optimize detection of benefits and mitigate potential harms. Institutional review boards mandate a systematic assessment of risks and benefits before the onset of the trial to assure adherence to the principle of beneficence.

A potential harm from a randomized controlled trial is the random allocation itself. If researchers believe the test treatment is superior to the control treatment, then it is unethical to deny test treatment to the participants randomly assigned to the control group. Likewise, it is unethical to initiate or continue test treatment if researchers believe the control treatment is superior. The ethical conduct of randomized controlled trials requires researchers to have genuine uncertainty about the preferred treatment. The state of uncertainty has been called therapeutic equipoise. A related concept, clinical equipoise, "requires that there exist a state of honest, professional disagreement in the community of expert practitioners as to the preferred treatment…" [14]. Institutional review boards may require researchers to demonstrate equipoise before the initiation of a randomized controlled trial.

Ethicists define equipoise in terms of uncertainty about a difference between test and control treatments. How does the researcher know when equipoise no longer exists? One way is to test the null hypothesis of the randomized controlled trial. In superiority trials, the statistician defines the null hypothesis as the absence of difference between test and control treatments. The purpose of statistical tests is to use data accumulated in the trial to reject the null hypothesis and accept the alternative hypothesis by inference. When sufficient data exist to reject the null hypothesis, then the researcher may infer that one treatment is superior to the other and leave the state of equipoise.

Equipoise that exists at the beginning of a randomized controlled trial may not last for the entire duration of the trial. Sometimes contemporaneous trials elsewhere in the world demonstrate the superiority of the test or the control treatment. Sometimes interim analyses of data generated within the randomized controlled trial reveal more-than-expected efficacy or harm. Whenever the researcher deviates from the state of equipoise, randomized allocation must stop. The researcher has a fiduciary duty to offer participants the treatment proven to be superior. Institutional review boards may require external review of accumulating data from a randomized controlled trial to judge the ongoing status of equipoise. The external review is performed by a data and safety monitoring board (DSMB), a group made up of independent experts who have no conflicts of interest with the conduct of the randomized controlled trial. The DSMB has multiple roles to safeguard the well-being of study participants and ensure the scientific integrity of the trial. The roles of the DSMB include reviewing data from inside and outside the trial and then recommending the continuation or curtailment of the trial [15].

Ethical Considerations Related to Comparative Effectiveness Trials

It is common to use placebos in randomized controlled trials to establish the efficacy of a new intervention. The scientific rationale for a placebo control is also persuasive in the setting of comparative effectiveness studies if there is a small effect size for the usual care treatment [23]. In some situations, the use of placebos in comparative effectiveness trials may be unethical if a previous placebo-controlled trial demonstrated a reduction in mortality, irreversible morbidity, or serious adverse events [9].

A case study illustrates the ethical use of placebos in trials. The Systolic Hypertension in the Elderly Program (SHEP) was a randomized, placebo-controlled trial in elderly patients with systolic hypertension. In SHEP, the test antihypertensive treatment, chlorthalidone, demonstrated a significant reduction in non-fatal myocardial infarction or coronary heart disease death when compared to the placebo [17]. The SHEP study was followed by the comparative effectiveness trial named ALLHAT. In ALLHAT, chlorthalidone was the active control treatment [7]. Because of the benefits of chlorthalidone demonstrated in SHEP, a placebo comparison was not ethically feasible in ALLHAT [16].

Investigators face additional ethical questions in the design of comparative effectiveness studies. Sometimes the intervention is directed at the health-care provider, but the outcome is measured in the patient. Examples occur with research designed to test interventions to reduce hospital readmissions: the discharging physician or nurse or pharmacist may receive the intervention while the readmission outcome is measured at the patient level. The ethical question is, "Who is the research participant and who should give consent?" Ethical questions are further complicated when the patient is a member of a vulnerable class, for example, a prisoner. None of these questions have simple answers and all require thoughtful consideration during the design of comparative effectiveness studies [22].

If randomized controlled trials have already established the efficacy of an intervention, then why pursue randomized controlled trials of effectiveness?

Efficacy and effectiveness trials are designed to answer different questions. Efficacy trials are explanatory, and they respond to the question, "Does the test intervention work under ideal conditions?" Effectiveness trials are pragmatic and answer the question, "How well does the test intervention work in real-world settings and in comparison with alternative interventions?" [21].

The results of efficacy trials may inform decisions by some users but not others. Regulatory authorities, like the United States Food and Drug Administration (FDA), use results from efficacy studies to approve and label new drugs and devices. Consumers, clinicians, purchasers, and policy makers use comparative effectiveness research to make informed decisions to improve health care for individuals and populations [13]. Efficacy studies that satisfy the regulatory requirements of the FDA do not necessarily prove that new drugs or devices are superior to currently available alternative therapies. Purchasers of health care have perspectives different from those of the FDA. Health insurance companies, Medicare, Medicaid, and other purchasers find efficacy studies to be necessary, but not sufficient, evidence to inform reimbursement decisions. Purchasers seek information from comparative effectiveness studies in order to limit reimbursement to treatments that optimize clinical and economic value.

What are the characteristics of randomized controlled trials that are designed for efficacy versus comparative effectiveness?

The characteristics that distinguish efficacy and effectiveness trials appear in Table 2.3. When compared with efficacy trials, effectiveness trials have fewer exclusion criteria, more active comparison groups, and greater participant diversity. In efficacy trials, the primary outcome may be a surrogate or clinical endpoint. To ascertain the primary efficacy outcome, research personnel may require specialized training or perform procedures that are not customary in usual clinical care. In effectiveness trials, the primary outcome is objectively measured, clinically relevant, and patient focused. The primary effectiveness outcome is detectable in the usual care setting without special tests or training [24].

Table 2.3 Differences between randomized controlled clinical trials to establish efficacy versus effectiveness

Efficacy trials of test intervention	Effectiveness trials of test intervention
Designed to establish the existence of a treatment effect under optimal conditions	Designed to establish whether treatment effects identified in efficacy trials carry over to more typical use of the intervention in clinical practice
Compare treatment effects of test intervention versus placebo or limited choice of comparators	Compare treatment effects of test intervention versus usual care or best available alternative therapy
Inclusion criteria designed to enroll a homogeneous sample of participants	Inclusion criteria designed to broadly define a heterogeneous group of participants who would likely receive the intervention in clinical practice
Inclusion criteria designed to enroll participants with the highest risk for the primary endpoint and highest likelihood to respond to the test intervention	Inclusion criteria designed to enroll participants with heterogeneous risks and responses
Exclusion criteria designed to yield homogeneous samples of participants with minimal comorbidities	Exclusion criteria are minimized to produce heterogeneous samples that represent the typical participants with comorbidities encountered in clinical practice
Exclusion criteria designed to minimize number of participants with low adherence	Exclusion criteria ignore adherence
Conducted by investigators with research and clinical expertise	Conducted by investigators with variable expertise
Conducted in research settings where adherence to clinical protocol is optimized	Conducted in usual practice settings where adherence to clinical guideline is variable
Conducted for shorter periods than those ultimately used in general patient care	Conducted for longer periods that approximate use in general patient care
Protocol for the test intervention is relatively inflexible	The clinician has greater flexibility to adjust the test and control interventions to the participant's circumstances and preferences
Follow-up for outcome assessment and intervention adherence may be more frequent and have more data collection than would occur in routine clinical practice	Follow-up for outcome assessment and intervention adherence will have frequencies and data collection requirements that mirror routine clinical practice
Auditors measure and optimize adherence to the research protocol by the investigators and study site personnel	There are no special strategies outside of routine clinical practice to monitor or improve adherence by research personnel

Table 2.3 suggests a clear distinction between efficacy and effectiveness trials. In reality, the distinction is less clear. Some trials have efficacy (explanatory) characteristics in some domains and effectiveness (pragmatic) characteristics in other domains. Clinical trial experts have created a tool to help researchers design and interpret trials that have overlapping features. The tool is called a Pragmatic Explanatory Continuum Indicator Summary (PRECIS) [24].

What are the statistical considerations in the design of comparative effectiveness trials?

The characteristics of efficacy trials tend to optimize homogeneity and minimize between-subject variance in the treatment groups. In contrast, effectiveness trials tend to have greater heterogeneity and larger variance. When variance goes up, statistical power usually goes down. To compensate for the loss of statistical power, effectiveness trials tend to require larger sample sizes than efficacy trials [21].

Comparative effectiveness trials may test hypotheses about differential outcomes associated with subpopulations or comorbidities. To detect interaction effects between participant characteristics and outcome, trials must have sufficient numbers of participants with the characteristic in question. The consequence to the trial design is a larger overall sample size [21].

In many randomized controlled trials, the unit of allocation is the participant. Sometimes comparative effectiveness trials employ a design that randomly assigns groups or clusters of individuals. A pertinent example is research designed to test interventions to reduce hospital readmissions. Consider a trial that compares patient readmissions after a test or a control discharge process. Ten doctors are assigned randomly to use the test discharge process on their patients. Another ten doctors are assigned to the control process. The outcome, readmission, is measured at the patient level. The patients of a specific doctor are a cluster of individuals: the patients may be correlated with each other in ways that influence readmission but that are unrelated to the discharge intervention and more related to the doctor-patient interaction. The amount of correlation is called the intracluster (or intraclass) correlation coefficient. As a consequence of intracluster correlation, the effective sample size is less than the total number of individual patient-participants. In addition, the total variance of the outcome measurement increases in proportion to the intracluster correlation coefficient. To maintain statistical power, the sample size must be larger for a cluster randomized trial than an individually randomized trial [2].

Summary

Comparative effectiveness researchers use clinical trials to generate evidence. When observational studies yield biased results, the randomized controlled trial design can mitigate biases. Investigators who design randomized controlled trials must be mindful of ethical principles that may not pertain to observational studies. Randomized controlled trials may be designed to answer questions of efficacy, effectiveness, or both. Tools like PRECIS exist to help investigators design and interpret clinical trials that address efficacy and effectiveness.

References

1. ALLHAT Officers and Coordinators for the ALLHAT Collaborative Research Group. The Antihypertensive and Lipid-Lowering Treatment to Prevent Heart Attack Trial (2002) Major outcomes in high-risk hypertensive patients randomized to angiotensin-converting enzyme inhibitor or calcium channel blocker vs diuretic: the Antihypertensive and Lipid-Lowering Treatment to Prevent Heart Attack Trial (ALLHAT). JAMA 288(23):2981–2997
2. Campbell MK, Piaggio G, Elbourne DR, Altman DG, CONSORT Group (2012) Consort 2010 statement: extension to cluster randomised trials. BMJ 345:e5661
3. Chobanian AV, Bakris GL, Black HR et al (2003) The seventh report of the joint national committee on prevention, detection, evaluation, and treatment of high blood pressure: the JNC 7 report. JAMA 289(19):2560–2572
4. Lidz CW, Appelbaum PS, Arnold R, Candilis P, Gardner W, Myers S, Simon L (2012) How closely do institutional review boards follow the common rule? Academic Medicine 87(7): 969–74. doi: 10.1097/ACM.0b013e3182575e2e
5. Colburn WA (2000) Optimizing the use of biomarkers, surrogate endpoints, and clinical endpoints for more efficient drug development. J Clin Pharmacol 40(12 pt 2):1419–1427
6. Moher D, Hopewell S, Schulz KF, et al Consolidated Standards of Reporting Trials Group (2010) CONSORT 2010 Explanation and Elaboration: Updated guidelines for reporting parallel group randomised trials. J Clin Epidemiol 63(8):e1–37. doi: 10.1016/j.jclinepi.2010.03.004
7. Davis BR, Cutler JA, Gordon DJ et al (1996) Rationale and design for the Antihypertensive and Lipid Lowering Treatment to Prevent Heart Attack Trial (ALLHAT). ALLHAT Research Group. Am J Hypertens 9(4 Pt 1):342–360
8. Eisenstein EL, Lemons PW 2nd, Tardiff BE, Schulman KA, Jolly MK, Califf RM (2005) Reducing the costs of phase III cardiovascular clinical trials. Am Heart J 149(3):482–488
9. Ellenberg SS, Temple R (2000) Placebo-controlled trials and active-control trials in the evaluation of new treatments. Part 2: practical issues and specific cases. Ann Intern Med 133(6):464–470
10. Getz KA, Wenger J, Campo RA, Seguine ES, Kaitin KI (2008) Assessing the impact of protocol design changes on clinical trial performance. Am J Ther 15(5):450–457
11. Gluud LL (2006) Bias in clinical intervention research. Am J Epidemiol 163(6):493–501
12. Goldstein J (2008) Study found cheap blood pressure meds are best. No one cared. In: The Wall Street Journal. Dow Jones Company. Available via http://blogs.wsj.com/health/2008/11/28/study-found-cheap-blood-pressure-meds-are-best-no-one-cared/. Accessed 6 Sep 2015
13. Institute of Medicine (2009) Initial national priorities for comparative effectiveness research. National Academies Press, Washington, DC
14. Miller PB, Weijer C (2003) Rehabilitating equipoise. Kennedy Inst Ethics J 13(2):93–118
15. Dixon DO, Weiss S, Cahill K et al (2011) Data and safety monitoring policy for National Institute of Allergy and Infectious Diseases clinical trials. Clin Trials 8(6):727–735
16. Pressel S, Davis BR, Louis GT et al (2001) Participant recruitment in the Antihypertensive and Lipid-Lowering Treatment to Prevent Heart Attack Trial (ALLHAT). Control Clin Trials 22(6):674–686
17. Prevention of stroke by antihypertensive drug treatment in older persons with isolated systolic hypertension. Final results of the Systolic Hypertension in the Elderly Program (SHEP). SHEP Cooperative Research Group (1991) JAMA 265(24):3255–3264
18. Protection of human subjects; Belmont Report: notice of report for public comment (1979) Fed Regist 44(76):23191–23197
19. Rossouw JE, Anderson GL, Prentice RL et al (2002) Risks and benefits of estrogen plus progestin in healthy postmenopausal women: principal results from the women's health Initiative randomized controlled trial. JAMA 288(3):321–333
20. Savovic J, Jones HE, Altman DG et al (2012) Influence of reported study design characteristics on intervention effect estimates from randomized, controlled trials. Ann Intern Med 157(6):429–438

21. Selker HP, Oye KA, Eichler HG et al (2014) A proposal for integrated efficacy-to-effectiveness (E2E) clinical trials. Clin Pharmacol Ther 95(2):147–153
22. Sugarman J, Califf RM (2014) Ethics and regulatory complexities for pragmatic clinical trials. JAMA 311(23):2381–2382
23. Temple R, Ellenberg SS (2000) Placebo-controlled trials and active-control trials in the evaluation of new treatments. Part 1: ethical and scientific issues. Ann Intern Med 133(6):455–463
24. Thorpe KE, Zwarenstein M, Oxman AD et al (2009) A pragmatic-explanatory continuum indicator summary (PRECIS): a tool to help trial designers. CMAJ 180(10):E47–E57

Chapter 3
Observational Studies

Jaeyong Bae and Carl V. Asche

Abstract This chapter discusses the use of secondary databases in outcomes research. Secondary databases, such as administrative databases and clinical registries, complement randomized controlled trials (RCTs) by evaluating large sample populations with a broader scope.

Secondary databases are also relatively more feasible than RCTs due to lower costs and greater timeliness. While administrative databases are originally created with the purpose of medical billing and administrative services, clinical registries are collected to assess and improve quality and outcomes of care. Administrative databases used for health outcomes research include (1) hospital inpatient discharge data, (2) ambulatory visits data, (3) emergency department visits data, and (4) health insurance claims data for both private and public insurers. Clinical registries contain more detailed clinical information on diagnoses, treatments, and prescriptions than administrative databases.

Introduction

Health outcomes research studies the effects of health-care interventions, the health-care process, and the structure of the health-care delivery system. Outcomes research is conducted by two primary means: RCTs and observation studies using secondary data.

J. Bae, PhD (✉)
Public Health and Health Education Programs, School of Nursing and Health Studies, Northern Illinois University, DeKalb, IL, USA
e-mail: jaeyong.bae@niu.edu

C.V. Asche, PhD
Research Professor, Director of Center for Outcomes Research, Department of Pharmacy Systems, Outcomes and Policy, Affiliate Faculty, Center for Pharmacoepidemiology and Pharmacoeconomic Research, University of Illinois at Chicago College of Pharmacy, Chicago, IL, USA

Research Affiliate, Centre on Aging,
University of Victoria, Victoria, British Columbia
e-mail: cva@uic.edu

© Springer International Publishing Switzerland 2016
C. Asche (ed.), *Applying Comparative Effectiveness Data to Medical Decision Making: A Practical Guide*, DOI 10.1007/978-3-319-23329-1_3

RCTs, widely regarded as the "gold standard" for assessment of health-care intervention, guarantee excellent internal validity because random assignment of subjects to control and treatment groups helps to ensure that the only difference between groups is their exposure to the intervention. Despite their inherent advantage in internal validity, a major limitation of RCTs lies in lack of external validity or generalizability. RCTs collect data from a targeted population with specific clinical relevance, and the sample size is typically limited.

Observational studies using secondary databases may fill the gaps of RCTs and address the lack of generalizability by assessing large sample populations with a broader scope. In addition to its advantage of external validity, the secondary data analysis is more feasible than RCTs due to lower costs and greater timeliness.

The main purpose of this chapter is to overview the use of secondary databases in outcomes research and to introduce commonly used secondary databases.

Types of Secondary Databases

Two primary types of secondary databases used in outcomes research are administrative databases and clinical registries. An administrative database is originally created with the purpose of supporting medical billing and administrative services. In contrast to administrative data, clinical registries are collected to assess and improve quality and outcomes of care. Provider and hospital characteristics data such as the American Hospital Association's annual survey and area characteristics data such as Area Health Resources Files are also frequently used in outcomes research.

Administrative Database

Two main producers of administrative data are health insurers and government agencies. While health insurers create administrative databases such as health insurance claims data for their financial and administrative purposes, federal and state government agencies collect administrative data such as hospital discharge abstracts to track and monitor health-care utilization and outcomes. Types of administrative data used for health outcomes research include (1) hospital inpatient discharge data, (2) ambulatory visits data, (3) emergency department visits data, and (4) health insurance claims data for both private and public insurers.

Strengths and Limitations of Administrative Data

There are several advantages to using administrative data in health outcomes research. They are readily available, are feasible to obtain and analyze, and cover a large number of longitudinal cases with various clinical situations [1]. Since administrative data are already collected for their primary purposes such as medical billing and administration, they are relatively inexpensive to acquire and use. In addition, administrative databases allow for tracking patients and providers over time and assessing time trends because they are made up of population-based longitudinal data.

Limitations of using administrative databases stem from the fact that they are not collected for research purposes but for medical billing and administration. The two primary limitations are coding inaccuracy and lack of clinical detail. Records reported in administrative data lack clinical details, such as patients' comorbidity and severity of illness, for comprehensive risk adjustment and analysis. Inaccurate or incomplete coding of diagnoses and procedures in administrative data is another significant threat to internal validity.

Use of Diagnostic and Procedure Codes in Administrative Data

Administrative data contain information on diagnoses and procedures. Diagnoses and procedures are typically coded using the International Classification of Diseases, Ninth Revision, Clinical Modification (ICD-9-CM) classification system. ICD-9-CM diagnosis and procedure codes provide information on the condition of a patient and medical services delivered, respectively.

Comorbidities or chronic conditions of patients are used for risk adjustment in health outcomes research. However, in contrast to clinical data, administrative data do not report detailed clinical information regarding comorbidities and complications. This lack of information may be addressed by using comorbidity indexes. Two commonly used methods to identify comorbidities using administrative data are the Charlson index and the Elixhauser index [2, 3]. The Charlson Comorbidity Index contains 19 comorbidities, defined using ICD-9-CM diagnosis codes. It also provides weighed scores to predict mortality and other outcomes. As an alternative to the Charlson Comorbidity Index, Elixhauser and her colleagues developed a list of 30 comorbidities based on ICD-9-CM diagnosis and procedure codes.

In addition to comorbidities, complications or adverse events can be captured using diagnosis and procedure codes in administrative data. For example, the Agency for Healthcare Research and Quality (AHRQ) developed patient safety indicators (PSIs) to identify hospital complications and adverse events following surgeries, procedures, and childbirth [4].

Examples

Health-Care Utilization Project

The Healthcare Cost and Utilization Project (HCUP) is a set of health-care databases maintained by the AHRQ [5]. The HCUP is the largest encounter-level hospital administrative database with all-payer information in the United States.

It contains more than 100 clinical and nonclinical variables including principal and secondary diagnoses and procedures, patient demographics, admission/discharge status, total charges, length of stay, and information on the primary payer for each hospital stay.

The HCUP consists of a series of national and state-level databases: (1) the National Inpatient Sample, (2) the State Inpatient Databases, (3) the Nationwide Emergency Department Sample, (4) the State Emergency Department Databases, (5) the State Ambulatory Surgery and Services Databases, and (6) the Kids' Inpatient Database. The National Inpatient Sample (NIS) is a nationally representative database of US hospital inpatient discharges. It is a 20 % stratified sample of discharges from all US community hospitals, containing 7 million hospital stays each year. Each discharge record includes a specific weight, which enables the generation of national estimates of inpatient care utilization. The State Inpatient Databases (SID) are state-specific databases capturing all inpatient discharges for 47 participating states. The HCUP also includes other nationwide and state-specific databases of hospital-based emergency department visits (the Nationwide Emergency Department Sample and the State Emergency Department Database), ambulatory surgery and other hospital-based outpatient visits (the State Ambulatory Surgery and Services Databases), and pediatric inpatient visits (the Kids' Inpatient Database).

National Hospital Discharge Survey

The National Hospital Discharge Survey (NHDS) is a representative national sample of inpatient discharges from nonfederal short-stay hospitals, administered by the National Center for Health Statistics (NCHS) and the Centers for Disease Control and Prevention (CDC) [6, 7]. For example, the 2007 NHDS collected data for approximately 366,000 inpatient discharges from 422 hospitals, equivalent to a national estimate of 34.4 million discharges [7].

The NHDS contains information on patient demographic characteristics, principal and secondary diagnoses and procedures, length of stays, sources of payment, and patient discharge disposition. The NHDS uses multistage probability sampling procedures to allow for generating nationally representative estimates of inpatient services.

National Ambulatory Medical Care Survey and National Hospital Ambulatory Medical Care Survey

The National Ambulatory Medical Care Survey (NAMCS) and the National Hospital Ambulatory Medical Care Survey (NHAMCS) are representative national samples for ambulatory visits [8–11]. Both surveys are administered by the National Center for Health Statistics (NCHS) at the Centers for Disease Control and Prevention (CDC). NAMCS collects health-care data provided by nonfederal office-based physicians, whereas NHAMCS collects health-care data provided by nonfederal hospital outpatient departments (OPDs) and hospital emergency departments (EDs). Both NAMCS and NHAMCS contain information on patient demographic characteristics, health status (reason for visit, chronic conditions), physician and hospital characteristics (specialty, practice ownership, predominant payer model), and geographic characteristics. Both surveys use multistage probability sampling procedures to allow for generating nationally representative estimates of ambulatory medical care services in the United States.

Medicare Databases

Medicare is a federally funded program that provides health insurance coverage primarily for the elderly [12]. More than 97 % of persons aged 65 or older in the United States are covered by the Medicare program. All Medicare beneficiaries are entitled to coverage of acute care hospitalizations and stays in skilled nursing facilities (Part A), and most of the Part A beneficiaries also enroll in Part B, which covers physician, outpatient, and home health services. The Centers for Medicare & Medicaid services (CMS), which administers Medicare, collects and maintains claims records of inpatient and outpatient visits for Medicare beneficiaries.

Medicare claims include diagnosis and procedure codes as well as beneficiary, physician, and facility identifiers, which enable researchers to track health-care utilization and outcomes across multiple providers. Primarily based on claims records, CMS constructs and houses a variety of administrative databases available to health services researchers [13]. One example of these databases is the Medicare Provider Analysis and Review (MEDPAR) file containing claims records for inpatient hospital and skilled nursing facility stays for fee-for-service Medicare beneficiaries [14].

Medicaid Databases

Medicaid is a joint federal-state program that pays for health-care services for the poor and the disabled. Medicaid is administered by individual states with federal oversight by CMS. Medicaid claims data is a unique and crucial resource to assess health-care utilization and outcomes of underserved groups such as racial and ethnic minorities, low-income people, and people living with disabilities.

Medicaid databases are obtained from either CMS or individual states. CMS collects Medicaid eligibility and claims data reported by individual states through the Medicaid Statistical Information System (MSIS) [15]. Several databases, including

Medicaid Analytic eXtract (MAX) data, are extracted from the MSIS [16]. The MAX data are a set of beneficiary-level data files containing information on eligibility, demographics, and claims for inpatient care, long-term-care, and other services including ambulatory care and prescription drugs [17]. State-specific Medicaid claims data are also available through individual states.

MarketScan Databases

The Truven Health MarketScan Commercial Claims and Encounters database is a proprietary database that contains enrollment information and claims data for inpatient care, outpatient care, and drug prescriptions from large self-insured employers [18]. There are several advantages of using the MarketScan claims database in outcomes research [19]. First, the MarketScan database captures a full spectrum of care including inpatient services, ambulatory care services, and drug prescriptions. The database also enables researchers to track patients across health plans over multiple years. Finally, the MarketScan database contains comprehensive information on outpatient prescriptions to track drug use patterns and prescription trends.

Clinical Registries

Clinical registries are collected to identify patients with particular diseases and conditions, track clinical practice patterns and outcomes, and improve quality and outcomes of care. They contain more detailed clinical information on diagnoses, treatments, and prescriptions than administrative databases.

Strengths and Limitations of Clinical Registries

Clinical registries are more appropriate for outcomes research than administrative databases are because the data are collected for the purpose of quality measurement and improvement. They are also considered as the most effective resources to measure quality of care and assess effectiveness of interventions. Data derived from clinical registries have advantages in completeness and accuracy compared to administrative databases. Clinical registries also have limitations. Clinical registries are more burdensome and costly to collect than administrative databases. In addition, they are generally focused on specific conditions or populations.

Examples

Surveillance, Epidemiology, and End Results (SEER) Program

The Surveillance, Epidemiology, and End Results (SEER) Program is a population-based cancer registry maintained by the National Cancer Institute, representing 28 % of the US population [20]. The SEER Program registries contain data on patient demographics, primary tumor sites, stages of cancer, dates of cancer diagnosis, dates of death, and causes of death.

Provider Characteristic Data

American Hospital Association Annual Survey databases

The American Hospital Association (AHA) Annual Survey databases have more than 1,000 fields of data for over 6,000 hospitals representing all short-term general acute hospitals in the United States. They include demographic information, organizational structure, facilities and services, utilization data, community orientation indicators, physician arrangements, expenses, and staffing [21]. The AHA annual survey is linked to other administrative databases to provide information on hospital characteristics such as teaching status, ownership, number of beds, and rural/urban location.

American Medical Association Physician Masterfile

American Medical Association (AMA) Physician Masterfile contains current and historical information on all physicians in the United States [22]. Specifically, the AMA Physician Masterfile includes data including physician name, demographic information, address, history of prior locations, type of practice, and medical school information.

Area Characteristic Data

Area Health Resources Files

Area Health Resources Files (AHRF) data contain more than 6,000 variables for each of the nation's counties and are available from the Health Resources and Services Administration (HRSA) to link data on health facilities, health professions, measures of resource scarcity, population health status, area economic activity, health training programs, and socioeconomic and environmental characteristics of individual counties [23].

Dartmouth Atlas of Health-Care Data

The Dartmouth Atlas of Health Care database provides a variety of measures at different geographic levels, including state, county, hospital service area (HSA), and hospital referral region (HRR) [24]. Measures in the Dartmouth Atlas database include Medicare spending and mortality rates, variation in the care of surgical conditions, and health-care supply such as number of hospital beds and physicians by specialties.

Conclusion

Observational studies using secondary databases have been prevalently used in outcomes research due to their advantages in generalizability and feasibility. There are two primary types of secondary databases: administrative databases and clinical registries.

Provider/hospital characteristics data and area characteristics data are linked with administrative data or clinical registries to provide information on provider and area characteristics. There are numerous administrative and clinical registry data sets available with their own strengths and weaknesses. Thorough assessment of potential databases, considering their strengths and weaknesses, is necessary to conduct observational studies using secondary databases.

References

1. Iezzoni LI (1997) Assessing quality using administrative data. Ann Intern Med 127(8_Part_2): 666–674
2. Charlson ME et al (1987) A new method of classifying prognostic comorbidity in longitudinal studies: development and validation. J Chronic Dis 40(5):373–383
3. Elixhauser A et al (1998) Comorbidity measures for use with administrative data. Med Care 36(1):8–27
4. Agency for Healthcare Research and Quality (2006) Patient safety indicators. [cited 28 Nov 2014]. Available from: http://www.qualityindicators.ahrq.gov/Downloads/Modules/PSI/V30/2006-Feb-PatientSafetyIndicators.pdf
5. Healthcare Cost and Utilization Project (2014) Databases. [cited 30 Nov 2014]. Available from: http://www.hcup-us.ahrq.gov/databases.jsp
6. Centers for Disease Control and Prevention (2014) National hospital discharge survey. [cited 30 Nov 2014]. Available from: http://www.cdc.gov/nchs/nhds.htm
7. Hall MJ et al (2010) National hospital discharge survey: 2007 summary. Natl Health Stat Rep 2010(29):1–20

8. Hing E et al (2010) National hospital ambulatory medical care survey: 2007 outpatient department summary. Natl Health Stat Rep 2010(28):1–32
9. Hsiao C-J et al (2010) National ambulatory medical care survey: 2007 summary. Natl Health Stat Rep 2010(27):1–32
10. Niska R, Bhuiya F, Xu J (2010) National hospital ambulatory medical care survey: 2007 emergency department summary. Natl Health Stat Rep 2010(26):1–31
11. Schappert SM, Rechtsteiner EA (2011) Ambulatory medical care utilization estimates for 2007. Vital Health Stat 13 (169):1–38
12. Centers for Medicare and Medicaid Services (2014) Medicare. [cited 30 Nov 2014]. Available from: http://www.cms.gov/Medicare/Medicare.html?redirect=/home/medicare.asp
13. Centers for medicare and Medicaid Services (2014) Research, statistics, data & systems. [cited 30 Nov 2014]. Available from: http://www.cms.gov/Research-Statistics-Data-and-Systems/Research-Statistics-Data-and-Systems.html
14. Centers for Medicare and Medicaid Services (2014) Medicare Provider Analysis and Review (MEDPAR) file. [cited 30 Nov 2014]. Available from: http://www.cms.gov/Research-Statistics-Data-and-Systems/Files-for-Order/IdentifiableDataFiles/MedicareProviderAnalysisandReviewFile.html
15. Centers for Medicare and Medicaid Services (2014) Medicaid statistical information system. [cited 30 Nov 2014]. Available from:http://www.medicaid.gov/medicaid-chip-program-information/by-topics/data-and-systems/msis/medicaid-statistical-information-system.html
16. Centers for Medicare and Medicaid Services (2014) Medicaid Analytic eXtract (MAX) general information. [cited 30 Nov 2014]. Available from: http://www.cms.gov/Research-Statistics-Data-and-Systems/Computer-Data-and-Systems/MedicaidDataSourcesGenInfo/MAXGeneralInformation.html
17. Borck R, Zlatinov A, Williams S (2012) The medicaid analytic eXtract 2008 Chartbook. Mathematica Policy Research
18. Truven Health Analytics (2014) Marketscan research databases. [cited 30 Nov 2014]. Available from: http://truvenhealth.com/your-healthcare-focus/analytic-research/marketscan-research-databases
19. Hansen L, Chang S (2011) Health research data for the real world: the MarketScan databases. Truven Health Analytics Inc, Ann Arbor
20. National Cancer Institute (2014) Overview of the SEER program. [cited 30 Nov 2014]. Available from: http://seer.cancer.gov/about/overview.html
21. American Hospital Association (2014) AHA annual survey database. [cited 30 Nov 2014]. Available from: http://www.ahadataviewer.com/book-cd-products/AHA-Survey/
22. American Medical Association (2014) AMA physician masterfile. [cited 30 Nov 2014]. Available from: http://www.ama-assn.org/ama/pub/about-ama/physician-data-resources/physician-masterfile.page?
23. Health Resources and Services Administration (2014) Overview: Area Health Resources Files. [cited 30 Nov 2014]. Available from: http://ahrf.hrsa.gov/overview.htm
24. Dartmouth Atlas of Health Care (2014) Atlas downloads. [cited 30 Nov 2014]. Available from: http://www.dartmouthatlas.org/tools/downloads.aspx

Chapter 4
Evaluating Published CER Evidence

Jinma Ren

Abstract It is challenging to translate the huge valuable information into practice in order to solve humanity problems of the world. From evidence to recommendation is a critical step to reach this goal. This chapter uses plenty of examples to introduce how to identify and assess evidence, how to evaluate recommendation's direction and strength, and how to develop a good recommendation in practice.

Aside from an instruction of evidence source and acquisition, this chapter also introduces the history of evidence level and provides an example of current modified evidence level for therapeutic studies.

Another highlight is that this chapter integrates a latest clinical practice guideline for preexposure prophylaxis (PrEP) with the details of developing an intervention recommendation based on the GRADE criteria. It could serve to guide other researchers to apply this procedure to develop other recommendations.

Introduction

Scientific information has surged around us along with developments in modern science and technology, especially in computing and the Internet that have dramatically improved the speed of information distribution. The number of articles in PubMed (Medline) published in 2013 was up to 1.1 million, over 13 times the number in 1950 (Fig. 4.1). However, a critical question simultaneously appears: how to translate this valuable research into practice in order to reach the ultimate goal of research that contributes to solving humanity's problems.

Moving from evidence to recommendation is an important step toward reaching the ultimate goal of research. The discovery of penicillin by Alexander Fleming in 1928 was an important landmark in the medical field, and its effective-

J. Ren, PhD
Center for Outcomes Research, Department of Internal Medicine, University of Illinois
College of Medicine at Peoria, Peoria, IL, USA
e-mail: jinmaren@uic.edu

© Springer International Publishing Switzerland 2016   37
C. Asche (ed.), *Applying Comparative Effectiveness Data to Medical Decision Making: A Practical Guide*, DOI 10.1007/978-3-319-23329-1_4

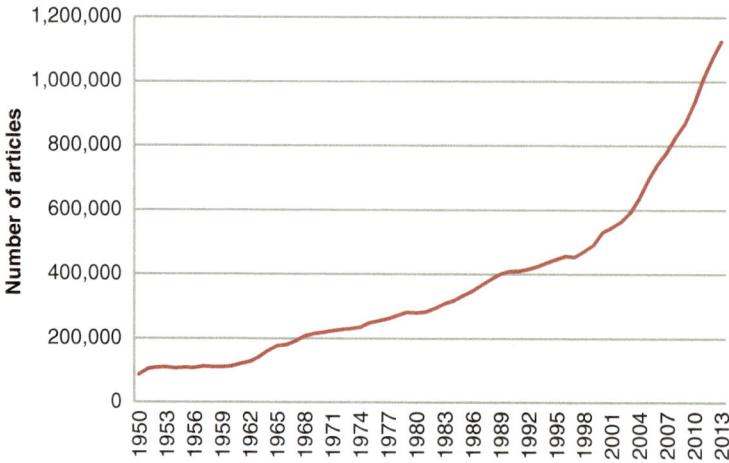

Fig. 4.1 The number of articles in PubMed (Medline) published every year (Data from http://dan. corlan.net/medline-trend.html)

ness against many previously serious diseases, such as bacterial infections caused by staphylococci and streptococci, has been applied to save countless lives throughout the world [1]. Another impressive example of translating evidence into recommendation is the eradication of smallpox. Smallpox, a deadly acute infectious disease, attacked about 50 million people annually due to without effective vaccination in the early 1950s. Only 10 years late, the epidemic fell by 70–80% because of the introduction of vaccination. Based on the evidence of vaccination's effectiveness, the World Health Organization (WHO) decisively made a recommendation to eradicate smallpox in 1967 and successfully reached this global goal in 1980 [2].

This chapter will discuss how to select relevant evidence to make appropriate recommendations and will give several examples of current recommendations for high-risk individual screening and cancer screening.

Identifying and Assessing Evidence

What Sort of Evidence?

Evidence is most commonly thought of as proof supporting an assertion. Identifying the questions of interest will help set the boundaries for relevant evidence, which is usually published in scientific literature such as professional journals, books, and/or government reports. For example, the question of the efficacy of condom use on HIV/AIDS prevention indicates that randomized controlled intervention trials should be searched, while the question of association between smoking and cancer indicates that prospective observational studies should be sought.

Where to Get Evidence?

A literature review is most frequently used to gather the evidence. After a question of interest is conceived, the first recommended step is to search the suitable recent systematic reviews that have already been published. It could be considered as a shortcut compared to conducting a new systematic review. For instance, Cochrane systematic reviews have been used widely recently [3, 4], but the risk of biased reporting in Cochrane systematic reviews also needs to be noted [5]. Of course, a new systematic review is definitely appropriate if the existing systematic reviews are old or fail to match the scope of the search strategy very well.

If a current systematic review is not available, a computer search of PubMed and Embase is usually the first step in looking for evidence based on certain search strategies tailored to appropriate types of studies, such as randomized controlled trials (RCT). For example, it appears that a new HIV prevention strategy, preexposure prophylaxis (PrEP), is "a way for people who do not have HIV but who are at substantial risk of getting it to *prevent* HIV infection by taking a pill every day" according to a definition from the Centers for Disease Control and Prevention (CDC). The US Public Health Service might not have found an existing systematic review to prove the efficacy of PrEP before it released the first comprehensive clinical practice guidelines for PrEP on May 14, 2014. So researchers searched the literature and found sufficient evidence based on several clinical trials that have demonstrated safety [6] and a substantial reduction in the rate of HIV acquisition for men who have sex with men (MSM) [7], men and women in heterosexual HIV-discordant couples [8], injection drug users [9], and heterosexual men and women recruited as individuals [10] who were prescribed daily oral PrEP with tenofovir disoproxil fumarate (TDF) and/or emtricitabine (FTC).

Checking references in articles also could yield additional relevant articles that were not identified by the computer search. Consulting experts in the field could get some evidence that has not yet been published and helps ensure that there are no obvious omissions from the literature review. If possible, additional search strategies also could be tried, such as searches for articles published in languages other than English, hand-searching relevant journals, and searching for unpublished material.

Accessing and Summarizing Evidence

Once studies have been identified based on a search strategy (such as outcome and study design), the relevance to the questions of interest should be addressed. Generally, using explicit rather than implicit criteria should improve the reliability of the process. The Grading of Recommendations Assessment, Development, and Evaluation (GRADE) system is a tool to rate the quality of evidence [11]. The GRADE process suggests that the quality of evidence should be rated as high, moderate, low, or very low based on study design, risk of bias, inconsistency, indirectness, imprecision, publication bias, large effect, dose response, and other issues (Fig. 4.2) [11–19]. The high-quality rating is defined as "further research is very unlikely to change our confidence in the estimate of effect"; a moderate quality ranking is defined as "further research is likely to have an important impact on our confidence in the estimate of effect and may change the estimate"; a low quality rating is defined as "further research is very likely to have an important impact on our confidence in the estimate of effect and is likely to change the estimate"; and a very low quality rating means "any estimate of effect is very uncertain" [20].

Summarizing the results of studies that have been identified is often possible and beneficial. Meta-analysis is one common summarizing method that focuses on contrasting and combining results from different studies in the hope of identifying patterns among study results, sources of disagreement among those results, or other interesting relationships that may come to light in the context of multiple studies [21]. Meta-analyses are often, but not always, important components of a systematic review procedure. The conclusion of a meta-analysis is statistically stronger than the analysis of any single study, due to increased numbers of subjects, greater diversity among subjects, or accumulated effects and results.

Study design	Quality of evidence	Lower if	Higher if
Randomized trial →	High	Risk of bias -1 Serious -2 Very serious	Large effect +1 Large +2 Very large
	Moderate	Inconsistency -1 Serious -2 Very serious	Dose response +1 Evidence of a gradient All plausible confounding
Observational study →	Low	Indirectness -1 Serious -2 Very serious	+1 Would reduce a demonstrated effect or +1 Would suggest a
	Very low	Imprecision -1 Serious -2 Very serious	spurious effect when results show no effect
		Publication bias -1 Likely -2 Very likely	

Fig. 4.2 Quality assessment criteria (Adapted from Guyatt et al. [11])

Evidence Level

The levels of evidence were first described in a report by the Canadian Task Force on the Periodic Health Examination in 1979 [22]. The report's purpose was to develop recommendations on the periodic health exam and base those recommendations on evidence in the medical literature. The authors developed a system for rating evidence when determining the effectiveness of a particular intervention (Fig. 4.3). At least one RCT with proper randomization was rated as the highest

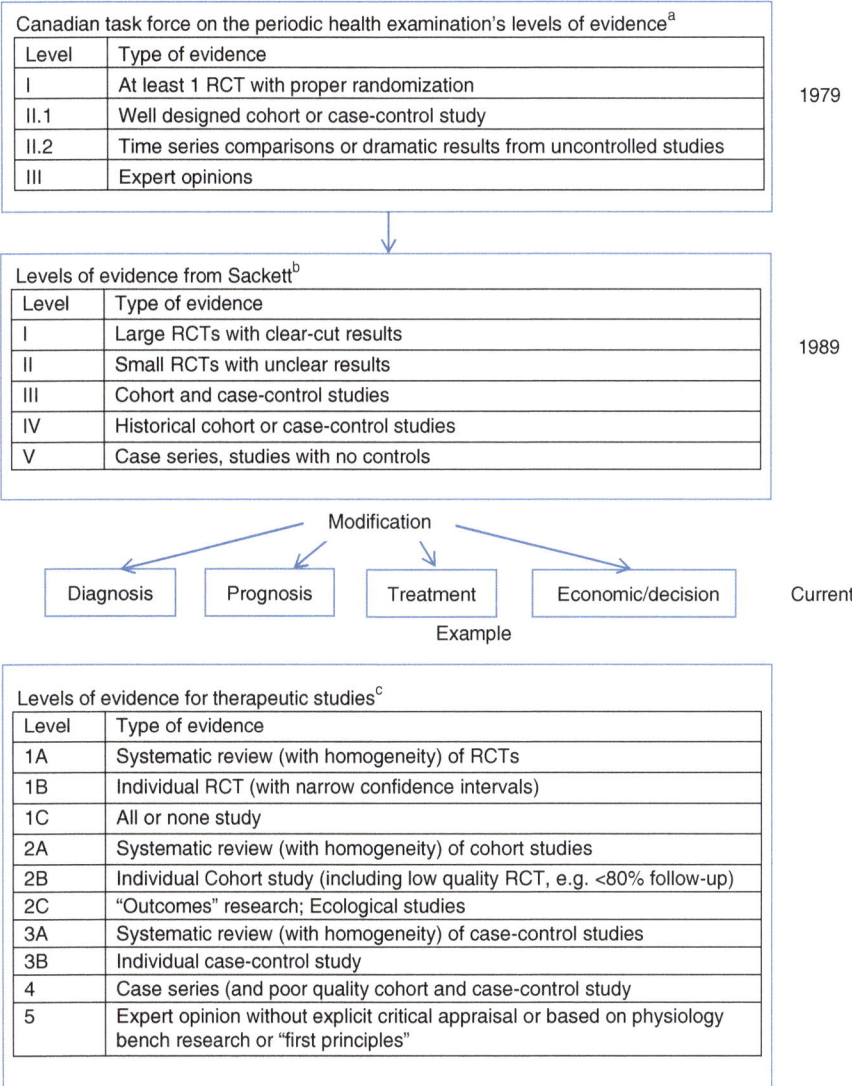

Fig. 4.3 Evidence rating system ([a]Adapted from "The periodic health examination [22]. [b]Adapted from Sackett [23]. [c]Adapted from CEBM [24])

level of evidence. Later, the levels of evidence were improved by Sackett in 1989 [23], who included five categories. Small RCTs with unclear results were downgraded into the second level. The levels of evidence have now been modified in order to fit different needs because diverse specialties are often asking different questions. As Fig. 4.3 depicted, the levels of evidence for treatment could be a little bit different from that for prognosis, diagnosis, and economic/decision analysis [24]. But systematic review (with homogeneity) of high-quality studies is always on the top of the pyramid of levels of evidence, while expert opinion without explicit critical appraisal, or based on physiology, bench research, or "first principles," is considered as the bottom.

Recommendations' Direction and Strength

A recommendation could offer a particular treatment, a routine screening/surveillance guideline, or a professional report to patients, health providers, ordinary people, or a government. Clinical guidelines are usually needed for some thorny diseases, such as cancers, because their diagnoses and treatments are very complicated. Clinicians can easily offer treatments to their patients with little or no hesitation based on the guidelines. Health departments can resolutely make a decision to raise a warning level for an infectious disease based on a surveillance report. On August 13, 2014, the CDC raised its travel warning to Level 3 (avoid nonessential travel), based on the outbreak of Ebola in Guinea, Liberia, and Sierra Leone, because it is the largest outbreak of Ebola in history and at least three Americans have been infected.

The GRADE guidelines have identified six determinants of the direction and strength of recommendations, including the estimated magnitude of the effect of the interventions on important outcomes, confidence in those estimates, estimates of typical values and preferences, confidence in those estimates, variability of values and preferences, and resource use. Moreover, as Table 4.1 shows, the six determinants have been summarized into four domains, namely, the balance between desirable and undesirable effects, the quality of evidence, values and preferences, and costs [25, 26].

Balance Between Desirable and Undesirable Effects

Large relative effects of an intervention/treatment consistently pointing in the same direction (toward desirable or toward undesirable effects) are more likely to warrant a strong recommendation. In contrast, large relative effects of an intervention/treatment pointing in opposite directions will lead to weak recommendations. Large absolute effects also contribute to a strong recommendation compared to small

Table 4.1 Domains that contribute to the strength of a recommendation

Factor	Comment
Balance between desirable and undesirable effects, with consideration of values and preferences	The larger the difference between the desirable and undesirable effects, the higher the likelihood that a strong recommendation is warranted. The narrower the gradient, the higher the likelihood that a weak recommendation is warranted
Quality of evidence: confidence in the magnitude of estimates of effect of the interventions on important outcomes	The higher the quality of evidence, the higher the likelihood that a strong recommendation is warranted
Values and preferences: confidence in values and preferences and variability	The more values and preferences vary, or the greater the uncertainty in values and preferences, the higher the likelihood that a weak recommendation is warranted
Costs: resource allocation and use	The higher the costs of an intervention—that is, the greater the resources consumed—the lower the likelihood that a strong recommendation is warranted

Adapted from:
Andrews et al. [26]
Guyatt et al. [27]

absolute effects because baseline risk can influence the balance of desirable and undesirable outcomes. For example, using low-dose aspirin for reductions in death and recurrent myocardial infarction could be a strong recommendation because of the very large gradient between the benefits and the undesirable consequences (minimal side effects) and costs.

Balancing the magnitude of desirable and undesirable effects requires considering the associated values and preferences; otherwise, it may be misleading. Ideally, best estimates of values and preferences are based on systematic reviews of relevant studies and clinicians' experiences with patients. Explicit, transparent statements of the panel's choices are imperative whatever the source of estimates of typical values and preferences.

Confidence in Best Estimates of Magnitude of Effects (Quality of Evidence)

Quality of evidence has been discussed in the above sections. Quality of evidence ratings are determined by eight criteria. The five that result in rating down the quality of evidence are risk of bias, inconsistency, indirectness, imprecision, and publication bias, whereas the remaining three criteria that lead to an increase in evidence quality are large magnitude of effect, dose–response gradient, and reduction of all plausible confounding.

Uncertainty and Variability in Values and Preferences

Panels often could be uncertain about typical values and preferences because systematic studies of patients' values and preferences are very limited [26]. The greater that uncertainty, the more likely it is that they will make a weak recommendation. On occasion, panels could be confident regarding a typical patient's values and preferences based on clinical experience. For instance, pregnant women's strong aversion to even a small risk of important fetal abnormalities may be one such situation [26, 27].

Large variability in values and preferences may also cause a weak recommendation. Under this circumstance, a single recommendation might be less likely to apply uniformly across all patients, and specific recommendations could be needed for specific patients.

Develop and Grade Recommendations

The above sections have discussed the identification and assessment of the evidence and the direction and strength of recommendations. However, the majority of readers could be more interested in how to develop and grade a recommendation in practice. Therefore, we briefly describe the procedure of developing a recommendation step by step below (also see a checklist in Table 4.2).

The first step should define the population, the intervention and the alternative, and the relevant outcomes. For instance, in order to develop a recommendation about preexposure prophylaxis (PrEP) for HIV prevention, we need to define that the population is people who do not have HIV but who are at substantial risk of getting it; that the intervention is to take a pill (brand name Truvada, which is used in combination with other medicines to treat HIV) daily when exposed to HIV through sex or injection drug use; and that the outcomes are the effective rate of HIV prevention, safety, and toxicity.

The second step is to collect and summarize the relevant evidence. As Table 4.2 depicted, we could start by assuming high quality if randomized trials are available, or we start by assuming low quality if only well-done observational studies are available. Then, we grade randomized trials down from high to moderate, low, or very low depending on their limitations, and we grade well-done observational studies up to moderate or even high depending on special strengths. Studies starting at very low, such as observational studies with limitations, will not be upgraded. Only observational studies with no threats to validity can be upgraded. Tables 4.3 and 4.4 are examples of applying GRADE

Table 4.2 A checklist for developing and grading recommendations

1. Define the population, the intervention and alternative, and the relevant outcomes
2. Summarize the relevant evidence (relying on systematic reviews)
If randomized trials are available, start by assuming high quality; if well-done observational studies are available, assume low quality, but then check for the following:
Serious methodological limitations (lack of blinding, concealment, high loss to follow-up, stopped early)
Indirectness in population, intervention, or outcome (use of surrogates)
Inconsistency in results
Imprecision in estimates
Grade RCTs down from high to moderate, low, or very low, depending on their limitations, or downgrade observational studies to very low
If no randomized trials are available but well-done observational studies are available (including indirectly relevant trials and well-done observational studies), start by assuming low quality, but then check for the following:
Large or very large treatment effect
All plausible confounders would diminish effect of intervention
Dose–response gradient
Grade up to moderate or even high depending on special strengths or weaknesses. Studies starting at very low will not be upgraded. Observational studies with limitations will not be upgraded. Only observational studies with no threats to validity can be upgraded
3. Decide on best estimates of benefits, harms, burden, and costs for relevant population
4. Decide on whether the benefits are, overall, worth the harms, burden, and costs for relevant population and decide how clear and precise this balance is

Adapted from Schunemann et al. [29]

criteria to collect and summarize evidence in order to develop the 2014 Clinical Practice Guideline for PrEP.

The next step is to estimate the benefits, harms, burden, and costs for the relevant population. The higher the costs of an intervention—that is, the greater the resources consumed—the lower the likelihood that a strong recommendation is warranted. Safety and toxicity are also evaluated for PrEP (Table 4.5) in order to balance the benefits and harms.

Finally, a decision will be made depending on whether the benefits are, overall, worth the harms, burden, and costs for the relevant population. We use the example of PrEP to further illustrate the final decision. As we all know, the human body cannot get rid of HIV, and no safe and effective cure currently exists, although scientists are working hard to find one and remain hopeful. Obviously, preventing HIV infection is the priority we should consider for making the decision. Moreover, strong evidence has shown that PrEP is effective in preventing HIV

Table 4.3 Evidence summary: overall evidence quality

| Study | Outcome analyses—HIV incidence (mITT) | | Effect—HR [efficacy estimate] (95 % CI) |
	Agent	Control	
iPrEx (MSM)	36 infections among 1224 persons	64 infections among 1217 persons	0.56 [44 %] (0.37–0.85)
US MSM safety trial	3 infectious among 201 persons (all 3 in delayed arm, not oil TDF)	4 infections among 199 persons (1 acute infection at enrollment)	Not reported
Partners PrEP (heterosexual men and women)	TDF 17 infections among 1572 persons; TDF/FTC 13 infections among 1568 persons	52 infections among 1568 persons	TDF / TDF/FTC — All: 0.33 [67 %] (0.19–0.56) / 0.25 [75 %] (0.13–0.45); Women: 0.29 [71 %] (0.13–0.63) / 0.34 [66 %] (0.16–0.72); Men: 0.37 [63 %] (0.17–0.80) / 0.16 [84 %] (0.06–0.46)
TDF2 (heterosexual men and women)	9 infectious among 601 persons; 1.2 infections/100 person-years	24 infections among 599 persons; 3.1 infections per 100 person-years	0.38 [62 %] (0.17–0.79)
FEM-PrEP (heterosexual women)	33 infections among 1024 persons; 4.7 infections per 100 person-years	35 infections among 1032 persons; 5.0 infections per 100 person-years	0.94 [6 %][a] (0.59–1.52)
West African trial (heterosexual women)	2 infectious among 427 persons; 0.86 infections per 100 person-years	6 infections among 432 persons; 2.48 infections per 100 person-years	0.35 [65 %][a] (0.03–1.93)
VOICE (heterosexual women)	TDF 52 infections among 993 persons; 6.3 infections per 100 person-years; TDF/FTC 61 infections among 985 persons; 4.7 infections per 100 person-years	35 infections among 999 persons 4.2 infections per 100 person-years	TDF 1.49 [−50 %][a] (0.97–2.3); TDF/FTC 1.04 [−4 %][a] (0.73, 1.5)
BTS (injection drug users)	17 infections among 1204 persons; 0.35 infections per 100 person-years	33 infections among 1207 persons; 0.68 infections per 100 person-years	0.51 [49 %] (9.6, 72.2)

Adapted from preexposure prophylaxis for the prevention of HIV infection in the United States—2014 clinical practice guideline

mITT modified intent to treat analysis, *HR* hazard ratio

[a]Not statistically significant

Table 4.4 Evidence summary: HIV incidence findings

Study	Design[a]	Participants Agent	Control	Limitations	Quality of evidence
Among men who have sex with men					
iPrEx trial	Phase 3	TDF/FTC (n = 1251)	Placebo (n = 1248)	Adherence	High
US MSM safety trial	Phase 2	TDF (n = 201)	Placebo (n = 199)	Minimal	High
Among heterosexual men and women					
Partners PrEP	Phase 3	TDF (n = 1589) TDF/FTC (n = 1583)	Placebo (n = 1586)	Minimal	High
TDF2	Phase 2	TDF/FTC (n = 611)	Placebo (n = 608)	High loss to follow-up: modest sample size	Moderate
Among heterosexual women					
FEM-PrEP	Phase 3	TDF/FTC (n = 1062)	Placebo (n = 1058)	Stopped at interim analysis, limited follow-up time; very low adherence to drug regimen	Low
West African trial	Phase 2	TDF (n = 469)	Placebo (n = 467)	Stopped early for operational concerns; small sample size: limited follow-up time on assigned drug	Low
VOICE	Phase 2B	TDF (n = 1007) TDF/FTC (n = 1003)	Placebo (n = 1009)	TDF arm stopped at interim analysis (futility); very low adherence to drug regimen in both TDF and TDF/FTC arms	Low
Among injection drug users					
BTS	Phase 3	TDF (n = 1204)	Placebo (n = 1207)	Minimal	High

Adapted from preexposure prophylaxis for the prevention of HIV infection in the United States—2014 clinical practice guideline

Note: GRADE quality ratings

High further research is very unlikely to change our confidence in the estimate of effect

Moderate further research is likely to have an important impact on our confidence in the estimate of effect and may change the estimate

Low further research is very likely to have an important impact on our confidence in the estimate of effect and is likely to change the estimate, *Very low* any estimate of effect is very uncertain

[a]All trials in this table were randomized, double-blind, prospective clinical trials

Table 4.5 Evidence summary: safety and toxicity

Study	Outcome analyses	
	Agent	Control
Grade 3/4 adverse clinical events[a]		
iPrEx	52 events	59 events
TDF2	9 events	10 events
West African trial	NR	NR
Grade 3/4 adverse laboratory events[a]		
iPrEx	59 events	48 events
TDF2	32 events	32 events
West African trial	1 event	5 events
Grade 3/4 adverse events (clinical and laboratory)[a]		
Partners PrEP	TDF: 323 events TDF/FTC: 337 events	307 events
FEM-PrEP	NR	NR
US MSM safety trial	36 events	26 events
VOICE	NR	NR
BTS	175 events	173 events

Adapted from preexposure prophylaxis for the prevention of HIV infection in the United States—2014 clinical practice guideline

NR not reported

[a]*RDBPCT* randomized, double-blind, prospective clinical trial

infection for a specific population, and it doesn't increase the likelihood of adverse events. Further, PrEP is covered by most insurance programs, and it also could be paid for by medication assistance programs if there is no insurance [28], which makes it possible for all target populations. Based on that information, the US Public Health Service released the first comprehensive clinical practice guidelines for PrEP on May 14, 2014.

However, it should be noted that every recommendation has its preconditions and requirements. As Table 4.6 shows, PrEP is not for everyone. People who use PrEP should have a substantial risk of acquiring HIV infection, satisfy clinical eligibility requirements, and comply with instructions regarding dosages and other services (such as follow-up visits every 3 months).

Table 4.6 Summary of guidance for PrEP use

	Men who have sex with men	Heterosexual women and men	Injection drug users
Detecting substantial risk of acquiring HIV infection	HIV-positive sexual partner Recent bacterial STI High number of sex partners History of inconsistent or no condom use Commercial sex work	HIV-positive sexual partner Recent bacterial STI High number of sex partners History of inconsistent or no condom use Commercial sex work In high-prevalence area or network	HIV-positive injecting partner Sharing injection equipment Recent drug treatment (but currently injecting)
Clinically eligible	Documented negative HIV test result before prescribing PrEP No signs/symptoms of acute HIV infection Normal renal function: no contraindicated medications Documented hepatitis B virus infection and vaccination status		
Prescription	Daily, continuing, oral doses of TDF/FTC (Truvada), $\leq$90-day supply		
Other services	Follow-up visits at least every 3 months to provide the following: HIV test, medication adherence counseling, behavioral risk reduction support, side-effect assessment, STI symptom assessment At 3 months and every 6 months thereafter, assess renal function Every 6 months, test for bacterial STIs		
	Do oral/rectal STI testing	Assess pregnancy intent Pregnancy test/every 3 months	Access to clean needles/ syringes and drug treatment services

Adapted from preexposure prophylaxis for the prevention of HIV infection in the United States—2014 clinical practice guideline

STI sexually transmitted infection

References

1. Fleming A (1980) Classics in infectious diseases: on the antibacterial action of cultures of a penicillium, with special reference to their use in the isolation of B. influenzae by Alexander Fleming, Reprinted from the British Journal of Experimental Pathology 10:226–236, 1929. Rev Infect Dis 2:129–139
2. Smallpox (2007) Accessed 10 Aug 2014, at http://web.archive.org/web/20070921235036/ http://www.who.int/mediacentre/factsheets/smallpox/en/

3. Ubbink DT, Santema TB, Stoekenbroek RM (2014) Systemic wound care: a meta-review of cochrane systematic reviews. Surg Technol Int 24:99–111
4. Brown J, Farquhar C (2014) Endometriosis: an overview of Cochrane Reviews. Cochrane Database Syst Rev 3:CD009590
5. Hopp L (2014) Risk of bias reporting in Cochrane systematic reviews. Int J Nurs Pract doi: 10.1111/ijin.12252
6. Grohskopf LA, Chillag KL, Gvetadze R et al (2013) Randomized trial of clinical safety of daily oral tenofovir disoproxil fumarate among HIV-uninfected men who have sex with men in the United States. J Acquir Immune Defic Syndr 64:79–86
7. Grant RM, Lama JR, Anderson PL et al (2010) Preexposure chemoprophylaxis for HIV prevention in men who have sex with men. N Engl J Med 363:2587–2599
8. Baeten JM, Donnell D, Ndase P et al (2012) Antiretroviral prophylaxis for HIV prevention in heterosexual men and women. N Engl J Med 367:399–410
9. Choopanya K, Martin M, Suntharasamai P et al (2013) Antiretroviral prophylaxis for HIV infection in injecting drug users in Bangkok, Thailand (the Bangkok Tenofovir Study): a randomised, double-blind, placebo-controlled phase 3 trial. Lancet 381:2083–2090
10. Thigpen MC, Kebaabetswe PM, Paxton LA et al (2012) Antiretroviral preexposure prophylaxis for heterosexual HIV transmission in Botswana. N Engl J Med 367:423–434
11. Guyatt G, Oxman AD, Akl EA et al (2011) GRADE guidelines: 1. Introduction-GRADE evidence profiles and summary of findings tables. J Clin Epidemiol 64:383–394
12. Guyatt GH, Oxman AD, Kunz R et al (2011) GRADE guidelines: 2. Framing the question and deciding on important outcomes. J Clin Epidemiol 64:395–400
13. Balshem H, Helfand M, Schunemann HJ et al (2011) GRADE guidelines: 3. Rating the quality of evidence. J Clin Epidemiol 64:401–406
14. Guyatt GH, Oxman AD, Vist G et al (2011) GRADE guidelines: 4. Rating the quality of evidence—study limitations (risk of bias). J Clin Epidemiol 64:407–415
15. Guyatt GH, Oxman AD, Montori V et al (2011) GRADE guidelines: 5. Rating the quality of evidence—publication bias. J Clin Epidemiol 64:1277–1282
16. Guyatt GH, Oxman AD, Kunz R et al (2011) GRADE guidelines 6. Rating the quality of evidence—imprecision. J Clin Epidemiol 64:1283–1293
17. Guyatt GH, Oxman AD, Kunz R et al (2011) GRADE guidelines: 7. Rating the quality of evidence—inconsistency. J Clin Epidemiol 64:1294–1302
18. Guyatt GH, Oxman AD, Kunz R et al (2011) GRADE guidelines: 8. Rating the quality of evidence—indirectness. J Clin Epidemiol 64:1303–1310
19. Guyatt GH, Oxman AD, Sultan S et al (2011) GRADE guidelines: 9. Rating up the quality of evidence. J Clin Epidemiol 64:1311–1316
20. Guyatt GH, Oxman AD, Vist GE et al (2008) GRADE: an emerging consensus on rating quality of evidence and strength of recommendations. BMJ 336:924–926
21. Greenland S, O'Rourke K (2008) Meta-analysis. In: Rothman KJ, Greenland S, Lash TL, eds. Modern Epidemiology 3rd ed., Philadelphia: Lippincott Williams, 652–682
22. The periodic health examination (1979) Canadian task force on the periodic health examination. Can Med Assoc J 121:1193–1254
23. Sackett DL (1989) Rules of evidence and clinical recommendations on the use of antithrombotic agents. Chest 95:2S–4S
24. Levels of evidence (2009) Accessed 18 Aug 2014, at http://www.cebm.net/oxford-centre-evidence-based-medicine-levels-evidence-march-2009/
25. Guyatt GH, Oxman AD, Kunz R et al (2008) Going from evidence to recommendations. BMJ 336:1049–1051

26. Andrews JC, Schunemann HJ, Oxman AD et al (2013) GRADE guidelines: 15. Going from evidence to recommendation-determinants of a recommendation's direction and strength. J Clin Epidemiol 66:726–735

27. Bates SM, Greer IA, Middeldorp S, Veenstra DL, Prabulos AM, Vandvik PO (2012) VTE, thrombophilia, antithrombotic therapy, and pregnancy: Antithrombotic Therapy and Prevention of Thrombosis, 9th ed: American College of Chest Physicians Evidence-Based Clinical Practice Guidelines. Chest 141:e691S–e736S

28. PrEP 101 (2014) Accessed 28 Aug 2014, at http://www.cdc.gov/hiv/basics/prep.html

29. Schunemann HJ, Jaeschke R et al (2006) An official ATS statement: grading the quality of evidence and strength of recommendations in ATS guidelines and recommendations. Am J Respir Crit Care Med 174(5):605–614

Chapter 5
Epidemiological Principles Applied to CER

Jinma Ren

Abstract Decision makers often struggle with how to make a decision to test everyone or not for a disease. As we all know, health-care decision making must be based on plenty of scientific evidences instead of gambling. On the other hand, any decision might have to take a certain risk because uncertainty always exists in the real world. The key question is how to understand and measure the risk of decision making.

This chapter starts from several relevant concepts in epidemiology, biostatistics, and health econometrics because these concepts are the foundation to understand the entire chapter, such as sensitivity, specificity, incidence, mortality, and cost. Then, this chapter discusses all determinants for testing everyone in detail. Furthermore, a practicable question tool is developed in order to help us make a quick decision on testing everyone or not.

Introduction

Health-care decision making is not gambling, so it must be based on plenty of scientific evidence. On the other hand, any decision might have to take a certain risk, because uncertainty always exists in the real world. For example, the US Preventive Services Task Force (USPSTF) recommends screening for colorectal cancer using fecal occult blood testing, sigmoidoscopy, or colonoscopy in adults, beginning at age 50 and continuing until age 75 [1]. It raises the question of why the USPSTF doesn't recommend the screening for all adults, because this recommendation definitely risks ignoring those who could get colorectal cancer at ages less than 50 years. To answer this question, we have to understand the risk of misclassification and know how to measure it.

Here, "to test everyone" is relative to a certain population. It doesn't mean to test anyone in the world. For instance, compared to the whole population, colorectal

J. Ren, PhD
Center for Outcomes Research, Department of Internal Medicine, University of Illinois
College of Medicine at Peoria, Peoria, IL, USA
e-mail: jinmaren@uic.edu

© Springer International Publishing Switzerland 2016   53
C. Asche (ed.), *Applying Comparative Effectiveness Data to Medical
Decision Making: A Practical Guide*, DOI 10.1007/978-3-319-23329-1_5

cancer screening for those aged 50–75 is not "testing everyone," but it also could be considered "testing everyone" when we only talk about this certain population whose ages are from 50 to 75.

This chapter will start from several relevant concepts in epidemiology, biostatistics, and health econometrics and then combine them with current recommendations to analyze why to test everyone or not. Although discussion about some definitions could be heavy and pedantic, it will help readers understand this chapter deeply.

Relevant concepts

Incidence and Prevalence

In epidemiology, incidence is the number of new cases in a particular period. It is often expressed as a ratio, in which the number of cases is the numerator and the population at risk is the denominator [2, 3]. When the denominator is the sum of the person-time of the risk population, it is also known as the incidence density rate or person-time incidence rate [4].

Prevalence is the number of cases (new and old cases) of a specific disease present in a given population at a certain time [2]. Unlike incidence measures, which focus on events, prevalence focuses on disease status. It is also named point prevalence, prevalence proportion, and prevalence rate.

The terms incidence and prevalence may be confused by researchers not familiar with epidemiology. In order to further elaborate on them, an example is in Fig. 5.1, including ten individuals who were observed during the period from January 1,

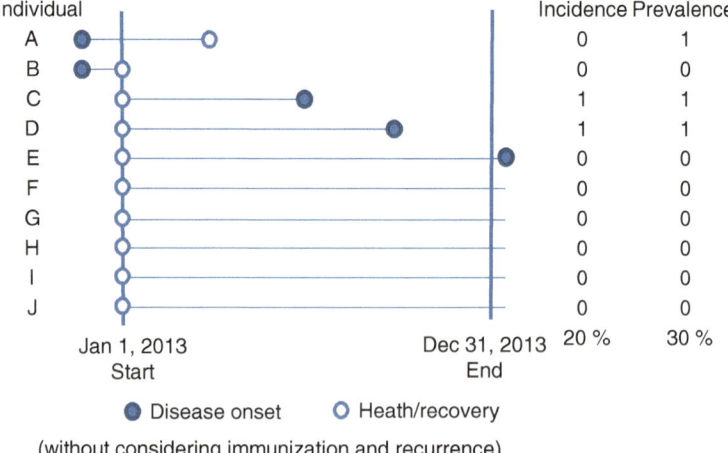

Fig. 5.1 Schematic diagram about incidence and prevalence

2013, to December 31, 2013. We assume all individuals were at risk (likely to have a disease, such as influenza). The individual *A* should not be counted for the incidence calculation because he/she was only previously a patient, whereas the individual *A* must be counted for the prevalence calculation. It is the critical difference about the numerator. Actually, it also appears as a subtle difference about the denominator. When some individuals have suffered from an uncured disease (such as hepatitis B), they should be excluded from the incidence calculation because they are not at risk of new infection any longer, but they could be included in the prevalence calculation.

If a disease could recur given a particular period, all onset events should be counted for incidence and prevalence calculations. So, it might not be surprising if an incidence or prevalence is greater than 100%.

Survival and Mortality

Survival is the length of time that a person lives after being diagnosed with a particular disease, such as colorectal cancer [2]. It is a major clinical parameter used to evaluate the efficacy of a particular therapy and the severity of a disease, and it is usually measured in "units" of 1 or 5 years. Survival rate curves are often used to compare the efficacy of a particular therapy (Fig. 5.2). On the other hand, mortality is the death rate, which reflects the number of deaths per unit of population in any

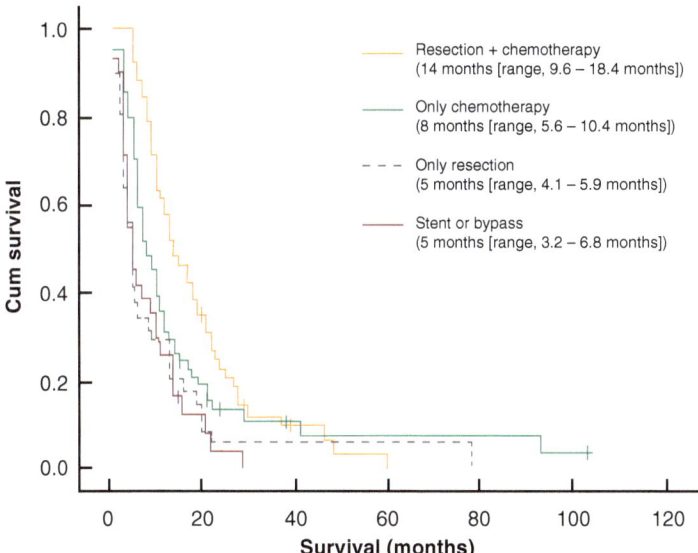

Fig. 5.2 Kaplan-Meier overall survival rate curve for patients with incurable stage IV colorectal cancer according to their initial management with resection and non-resection therapy (Adapted from Kim et al. [16])

specific region, age group, disease status, or other classification, usually expressed as deaths per 1,000, 10,000, or 100,000.

In order to measure disease burden, the quality-adjusted life year (QALY) is often applied in health economics and epidemiology because it reflects both the quality and the quantity of life lived. It assumes that a year of life lived in perfect health is worth 1 QALY (1 year of life × 1 utility value = 1 QALY) and that a year of life lived in a state of less than perfect health is worth less than 1.

Sensitivity and Specificity

Sensitivity and specificity are statistical measures of the performance of a binary classification test. They are often used to evaluate the efficacy of a test for clinical diagnosis or screening. Sensitivity measures the ability to catch true positives, so it is also called the true positive rate. In contrast, specificity measures the ability to catch true negatives, so it also called the true negative rate. For instance (Fig. 5.3), the sensitivity of the fecal occult blood screen test is the percentage of bowel cancer patients who are correctly identified as having bowel cancer (67%); the specificity of the fecal occult blood screen test is the percentage of healthy people (no bowel cancer) who are correctly identified as not having bowel cancer (91 %).

Generally, any test could present misclassification risk in the real world. As the upper part of Fig. 5.4 depicts, a cutoff selection must consider both sensitivity and specificity. If the cutoff line is moved toward the right in order to enhance the sensitivity, the specificity has to be weakened. Therefore, the receiver operating characteristic (ROC) curve is created to help find a point where both sensitivity and

		Patients with bowel cancer (as confirmed on endoscopy)		
		Condition positive	Condition negative	
Fecal occult blood screen test outcome	Test outcome positive	True positive (TP) = 20	False positive (FP) = 180	**Positive predictive value** = TP / (TP + FP) = 20 / (20 + 180) = **10 %**
	Test outcome negative	False negative (FN) = 10	True negative (TN) = 1820	**Negative predictive value** = TN / (FN + TN) = 1820 / (10 + 1820) ≈ **99.5 %**
		Sensitivity = TP / (TP + FN) = 20 / (20 + 10) ≈ **67 %**	**Specificity** = TN / (FP + TN) = 1820 / (180 + 1820) = **91 %**	

Fig. 5.3 Example of a binary classification test (Adapted from WIKIPEDIA [17])

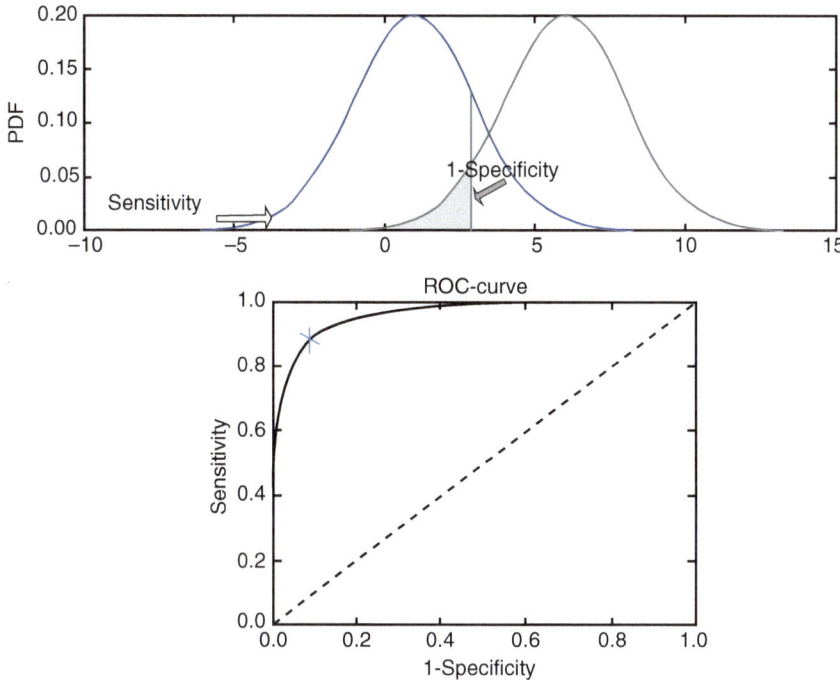

Fig. 5.4 Receiver operating characteristic (ROC) curve and sensitivity/specificity (Adapted from Haslwanter [18])

specificity reach the maximum possible. When drawing a top-left to bottom-right diagonal on the ROC diagram, the crosspoint with the ROC curve is the point we want (the "X" sign on the lower part of Fig. 5.4). The bigger the area under the ROC curve is, the better the effectiveness of a test would be.

The positive and negative predictive values (PPV and NPV, respectively) are also very important in screening and diagnostic tests. The PPV measures the ability to predict true positives, whereas the NPV measures the ability to predict true negatives. For example (Fig. 5.3), the PPV of the fecal occult blood screen test is the percentage of test-positive persons who really have bowel cancer (10 %); the NPV of the fecal occult blood screen test is the percentage of test-negative persons who really do not have bowel cancer (99.5 %). Obviously, the PPV and NPV are associated with the prevalence of a disease and the sensitivity and specificity of a test. As Fig. 5.5 depicts, given a fixed sensitivity and specificity, the PPV sharply goes up along with an increase in prevalence and just the opposite is true for the NPV. That's the reason why the PPV of fecal occult blood screen test for bowel cancer is very low (10 %) due to the low prevalence of bowel cancer. However, both PPV and NPV go up along with an increase in the sensitivity/specificity if the prevalence is fixed (Fig. 5.6).

Other derived measures include positive likelihood ratio (LR+), negative likelihood ratio (LR−), and diagnostic odds ratio (DOR). LR+ is the probability of a

Fig. 5.5 Relationship between the prevalence and the positive/negative predictive values given a fixed sensitivity (80 %) and specificity (90%)

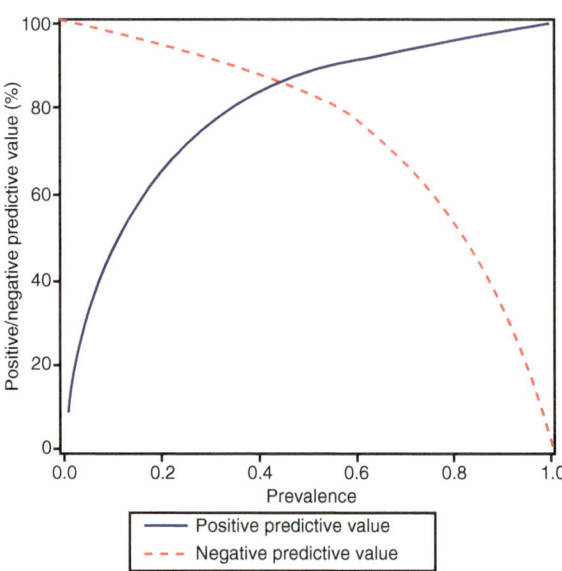

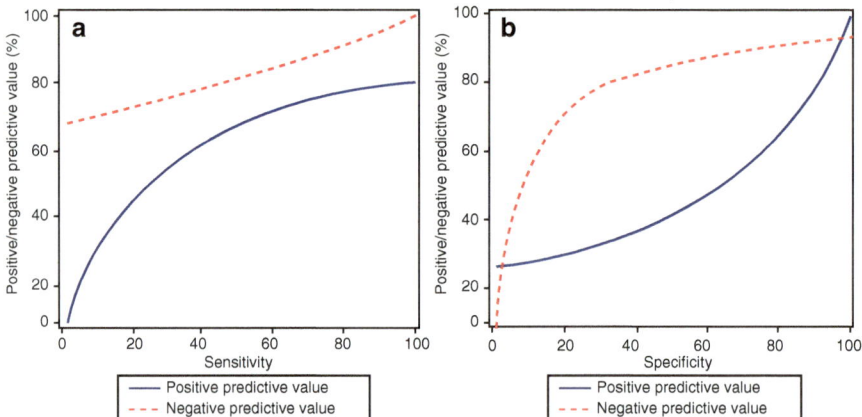

Fig. 5.6 Relationship between the sensitivity/specificity and the positive/negative predictive values: (**a**) prevalence = 30 % and specificity = 90 % and (**b**) prevalence = 30 % and sensitivity = 80 %

person who has the disease testing positive divided by the probability of a person who does not have the disease testing positive. LR− is the probability of a person who has the disease testing negative divided by the probability of a person who does not have the disease testing negative. DOR is defined as the ratio of the odds of the test being positive if the subject has a disease relative to the odds of the test being positive if the subject does not have the disease [5]. The definitions above can be obscure and unintelligible. But their calculations are very easy, according to the following formulas:

$$LR_+ = Sensitivity/(1-Specificity)$$
$$LR- = (1-Sensitivity)/Specificity$$
$$DOR = LR_+/LR-$$

Cost and Effectiveness

The terms mentioned above (such as incidence/prevalence and survival/mortality) might serve to measure an effectiveness or outcome, but they cannot reflect the other side (cost). Usually, we need to evaluate the cost before we scale up a screening in a population. The total cost includes fixed costs and variable costs. The fixed costs do not vary with the quantity of output in the short run (about 1 year). Examples include rent, equipment lease payments, and some wages and salaries, that is, costs that vary with time rather than quantity. Variable costs vary with the level of output. Examples include supplies, food, and fees for services [6].

Determinants for Testing Everyone

High Sensitivity and Specificity

High sensitivity and specificity are necessary for every test. Although we couldn't ideally expect both sensitivity and specificity to be 100 % in the real world, at least a reasonable level (such as >70 %) is needed for a diagnostic or screening test. If both sensitivity and specificity are very low (close to 50 %), the test should be discarded because it is more like throwing a coin to make a decision.

High Prevalence or Disease Burden

As previously discussed, the higher the prevalence is, the bigger the positive predictive value is if other conditions are fixed. That is to say, it is likely to be worth testing everyone if the prevalence of a disease is high. However, disease burden could be more important than prevalence. For example, a recent study reported that the prevalence of hemorrhoids in adults is very high (39 %) [7]. Hemorrhoids don't cause a heavy burden, so it is not at all necessary to examine everyone. In contrast, it is still worth testing everyone if a disease has a heavy burden, even if its prevalence is very low. The prevalence of human immunodeficiency virus (HIV) infection in adults in the United States is estimated to be only 0.6 % [8]; however, the heavy disease burden (low QALY, high mortality, and mental burden) of HIV has led to a new recommendation, released by the USPSTF recently [9], to screen all individuals aged 15–65 for HIV.

As Fig. 5.7 shows, cost must be also considered, although testing anyone could net great benefits if a disease has heavy disease burden and/or high prevalence. A country or state has to find a balance between the total cost and the benefits it may get before making a decision to test everyone for a disease. In the United States, a developed country, it is affordable to screen all individuals aged 15–65 for HIV. However, it might not be doable in developing countries and the third world, even if the prevalence of HIV is higher there.

Improvement of Prognosis

Improving a prognosis is also one of the important determinants for testing everyone. It would be useless to test everyone if a test couldn't improve the prognosis of a disease at all. For instance, rabies, a viral disease that causes acute inflammation of the brain in humans and other warm-blooded animals, is almost always fatal after neurological symptoms have developed in unvaccinated humans [10]. So screening or testing for rabies in a certain population loses its value because the patients with rabies couldn't get any benefit or very little benefit even if the disease is detected earlier. On the other hand, early detection could greatly improve the prognosis for some cancers (such as breast cancer and colorectal cancer), so that routine cancer screening could save many lives or at least improve the quality of life for cancer patients.

Culture

Aside from the evidence, decision makers also have to take into account the culture in a country or region before they make a decision to test for a disease or implement an intervention. The World Health Organization (WHO) and the Joint United Nations Programme on HIV/AIDS (UNAIDS) announced recommendations about male circumcision as HIV prevention in 2007 [11]. However, the Asian culture

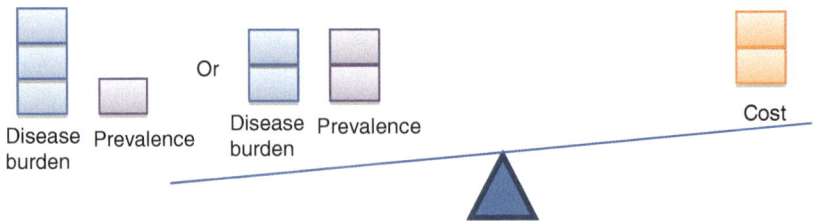

Fig. 5.7 Balance between benefit and cost for testing everyone

Table 5.1 Questions for making a decision to test everyone or not

Questions	Answers	Example (HIV)
1. Is the disease burden heavy (high incidence/prevalence, high mortality or mental burden)?	Yes	High mortality and metal burden
2. Is there a test (high sensitivity and specificity) for screening the disease?	Yes	HIV antibody tests: ELISA, rapid HIV test HIV antibody confirmation tests: Western blot, indirect fluorescent antibody
3. Can the early detection improve the prognosis of the disease?	Yes	Reduce risk for AIDS-defining events and death in persons with less advanced immunodeficiency and reduces sexual transmission of HIV [13]
4. Is it cost-effective to screening the disease?	Yes, in a certain population	More frequent testing is cost-effective for all risk groups [14]
5. Is the cost acceptable in the country/region?	Yes, in some countries/regions	Such as the United States
6. Does the culture in the country/region accept the disease screening?	Yes	Such as the United States
7. Can we make a decision to test everyone (or a certain population) now?	Yes	The US Preventive Services Task Force recommends to screen all patients aged 15–65 and other teens or older adults who are at an elevated risk for HIV infection [15]

leads to a barrier to accepting circumcision among the Asian people [12]. In Asia, people are not willing to do circumcision for themselves or their children, and sometimes they don't trust their doctors.

Feasibility

Feasibility for testing everyone could be considered as an integration of all determinants we have discussed above. That is to say, it would be infeasible if one of determinants is absent. Table 5.1 could help us comb through the questions (determinants) before a decision is made to test everyone for a disease.

References

1. Screening for colorectal cancer: U.S. Preventive Services Task Force recommendation statement (2008) Ann Intern Med 149:627–637
2. Medical dictionary (2014) Accessed 29 Aug 2014, at http://medical-dictionary.thefreedictionary.com

3. Rothman JK, Greenland S (1998) Modern epidemiology, 2nd edn. Lippincott-Raven, Philadelphia
4. Last JM, Spasoff RA, Harris SS (2001) A dictionary of epidemiology, 4th edn. Oxford University Press, New York
5. Diagnostic odds ratio (2014) Accessed 2 Sept 2014, at http://en.wikipedia.org/wiki/Diagnostic_odds_ratio
6. Drummond MF, Sculpher MJ, Torrance GW, O'Brien BJ, Stoddart GL (2005) Methods for the economic evaluation of health care programmes, 3rd edn. Oxford University Press, Oxford/New York
7. Riss S, Weiser FA, Schwameis K et al (2012) The prevalence of hemorrhoids in adults. Int J Colorectal Dis 27:215–220
8. List of countries by HIV/AIDS adult prevalence rate (2014) Accessed 2 Sept 2014, at http://en.wikipedia.org/?title=List_of_countries_by_HIV/AIDS_adult_prevalence_rate
9. Screening for HIV (2013) Accessed 4 Sept 2014, at http://www.uspreventiveservicestaskforce.org/uspstf/uspshivi.htm
10. Rabies (2014) Accessed 4 Sept 2014, at http://en.wikipedia.org/wiki/Rabies
11. WHO/UNAIDS announce recommendations about male circumcision as HIV prevention. Strategy should be employed with care (2007) AIDS Alert 22:66–67
12. Lau JT, Zhang J, Yan H et al (2011) Acceptability of circumcision as a means of HIV prevention among men who have sex with men in China. AIDS Care 23:1472–1482
13. Chou R, Selph S, Dana T et al (2012) Screening for HIV: systematic review to update the 2005 U.S. Preventive Services Task Force recommendation. Ann Intern Med 157:706–718
14. Lucas A, Armbruster B (2013) The cost-effectiveness of expanded HIV screening in the United States. AIDS 27:795–801
15. Moyer VA (2013) Screening for HIV: U.S. Preventive Services Task Force recommendation statement. Ann Intern Med 159:51–60
16. Kim SK, Lee CH et al (2012) Multivariate Analysis of the Survival Rate for Treatment Modalities in Incurable Stage IV Colorectal Cancer. J Korean Soc Coloproctol 28(1):35–41
17. WIKIPEDIA (2014) Sensitivity and specificity. Retrieved 2 Sep 2014, from http://en.wikipedia.org/wiki/Sensitivity_and_specificity
18. Haslwanter T (2014) Statistical data analysis. Retrieved 2 Sept 2014, from http://work.thaslwanter.at/Stats/html/statsTests.html

Chapter 6
The Question of Value

Minchul Kim, Carl V. Asche, and Inkyu K. Kim

Abstract This chapter discusses how to measure and evaluate the values in health-care decisions. The values of health-care decisions can be measured by health outcomes. The measured health outcomes are classified into clinical outcomes, humanistic outcomes, and economic and utilization outcomes. The clinical outcomes are the most commonly used health outcomes in comparative effectiveness research. However, evaluating the values of health-care decisions requires the economic and utilization outcomes (costs) also.

The values in health-care decisions can be evaluated to determine whether a health-care decision is an efficient use of society's resources. The economic evaluation methods are classified into the cost-health outcome evaluations and cost-only evaluations. The former included cost-effectiveness analysis, cost-utility analysis, cost-consequence analysis, and cost-benefit analysis, and the latter included cost-minimization analysis and cost-of-illness/cost-identification analyses.

The most common type of economic evaluation is the cost-effectiveness analysis (including cost-utility analysis) that compares the costs and outcomes of alternative approaches to reaching the "same" objective in order to determine which alternative accomplishes a given objective at the least cost. The cost-benefit analysis can compare widely varying programs and services with different outcomes to evaluate

M. Kim, PhD (✉)
Center for Outcomes Research, Department of Internal Medicine,
University of Illinois College of Medicine at Peoria, Peoria, IL, USA
e-mail: mchkim@uic.edu; cva@uic.edu

C.V. Asche, PhD
Research Professor, Director of Center for Outcomes Research, Department of Pharmacy Systems, Outcomes and Policy, Affiliate Faculty, Center for Pharmacoepidemiology and Pharmacoeconomic Research, University of Illinois at Chicago College of Pharmacy, Chicago, IL, USA

Research Affiliate, Centre on Aging, University of Victoria, Victoria, British Columbia
e-mail: cva@uic.edu

I.K. Kim, PhD
Battelle Memorial Institute, Atlanta, GA, USA
e-mail: ddz8@cdc.gov

© Springer International Publishing Switzerland 2016
C. Asche (ed.), *Applying Comparative Effectiveness Data to Medical Decision Making: A Practical Guide*, DOI 10.1007/978-3-319-23329-1_6

allocative efficiency among interventions between health care and other sectors. Cost-of-illness/cost-identification analyses estimate economic burdens of disease or treatment on society. Cost-minimization analysis identifies the least expensive alternative to minimize cost with an assumption of identical effectiveness.

Introduction

In a health-care delivery system, the value of a choice should be of greater concern to decision makers, patients, health-care providers, and governments. The value should define the framework for performance improvement in health care [1]. Health-care decisions, as well as prevention and intervention programs, are intended to protect people from diseases. Any preventive or treatment decision generates and enhances value for patients and other benefits to society.

Economics is the study of the optimal allocation of limited resources for the production of benefit to society, and it is therefore relevant to any health-care decision [2]. With scarce resources, a decision should be made to maximize net benefits of the health-care decision. The value of a health-care decision can be measured by costs and health outcomes. Health-care costs are an important issue to patients, health-care providers, third-party payers, and governments in making decisions about health-care practices. An economic evaluation determines whether an intervention is an efficient use of society's resources and can be defined as the comparative analysis of alternative courses of action in terms of both their costs and consequences [3].

Outcome Measurements

Health outcomes represent any change in patients resulting from medical care [4]. They are classified into three general categories: clinical outcomes, humanistic outcomes, and economic and utilization outcomes [5, 6]. The conceptual model of health outcomes is shown in Fig. 6.1.

Clinical Health Outcomes

Clinical outcomes are medical events resulting from disease or treatment [5, 6]. They are considered the most common outcomes in comparative effectiveness research [7]. Examples of clinical outcome measures include improved disease or symptom control, improved health outcomes and prescription medicine adherence, increased rates of vaccination or screening for disease, and an increase in patients' understanding and use of the health-care treatment. Multiple clinical outcomes may be selected for evaluation in a study when clinical aspects of interest exist in a target intervention [7].

Clinical outcomes are categorized into temporal aspect, objective assessments, composite endpoints, and intermediate endpoints [7]. The temporal aspects include

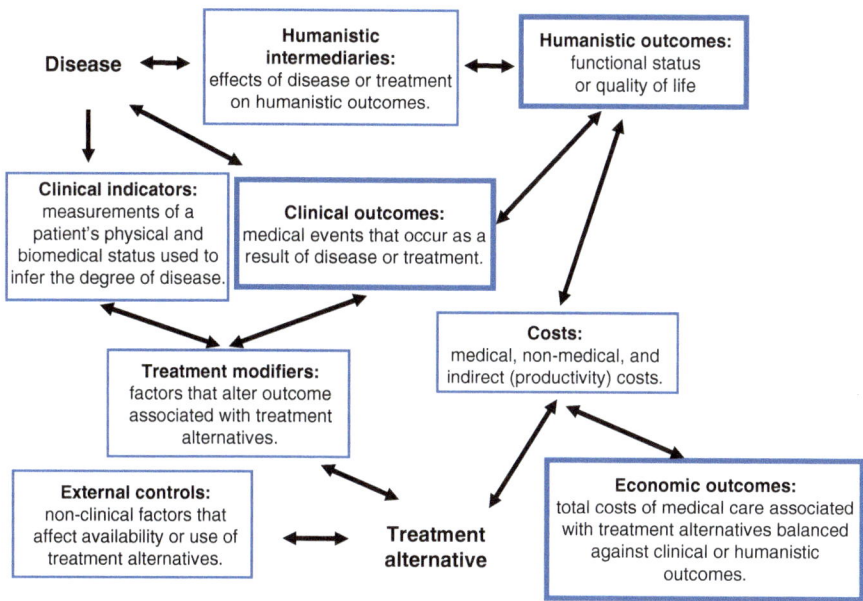

Fig. 6.1 The conceptual model of health outcomes: economic, clinical, and humanistic outcome (ECHO) model (Source: Kozma et al. [5])

incidence, prevalence, or recurrence of the condition of interest [7]. Objective measures, including mortality or lab tests, are those that are not likely to be changed by different health providers [7]. Composite or combined endpoints are measures composed of a series of component endpoints. In cardiology research, major adverse cardiac events (MACE) are the most commonly used composite endpoint [8]. Intermediate endpoints are biological markers for the condition of interest, such as the measure of serum lipids to reflect a reduction in coronary heart disease incidence and mortality [7].

Humanistic Outcomes

Humanistic outcomes are consequences of disease or treatment on the health status of patients [5]. They include measures of patient satisfaction, patients' quality of life, and daily functioning. The representative examples of humanistic outcomes are health-related quality of life (HRQL), patient-reported outcomes (PRO), and quality-adjusted life years (QALY).

HRQL is a broad-ranging multidimensional measure incorporating physical, mental, emotional, and social functioning [9]. It measures the effects of disease and treatment on the lives of patients [7, 10]. Patient information is obtained through questionnaires capturing the quality of life from the patient perspective. The current conceptualizations of HRQL include health status, functional status, quality of life, and sometimes social and economic stress [11].

PRO is any information on health outcomes provided by a patient without a physician's interpretation of the patient's response [11, 12]. In details, PRO includes a patient's ratings on several outcomes such as health status, health-related quality of life, quality of life, symptoms, functioning, and satisfaction regarding treatment [7].

QALY is a measure of health outcome assigning to each time period a numeric weight (from "0=death" to "1=perfect health") depending on the quality of life [3]. It combines the length of time and the quality of life (HRQL) of patients into one index as shown in Fig. 6.2 [13]. The length of time is based on the clinical outcome in question, such as mortality or life expectancy. The quality of life relies on utilities (ranging from 0 to 1) derived from economic and decision theory [7].

Utilities are estimated from the preference-based instruments where the preferences are based on the individuals' rating of their health states [7]. As instruments for rating individuals' health states, the standard gamble and time tradeoff methods [14, 15], the Health Utilities Index [16, 17], the EuroQol (EQ-5D) [18], the Short Form 6D (SF-6D) [19], and the Quality of Well-Being Scale are used [20].

In general, these instruments have from four to nine dimensions, each with three to six levels [13]. For instance, the EQ-5D has five dimensions in defining health states: mobility, self-care, usual activities, pain, and depression/anxiety [13]. Each dimension consists of three levels to classify a patient's health into one of 245 states [13].

Economic and Utilization Outcomes

Economic and utilization outcomes are health-care utilizations and costs, including direct, indirect, and intangible costs of medical treatments [5]. Economic outcomes represent the payer and societal perspective, while clinical outcomes and

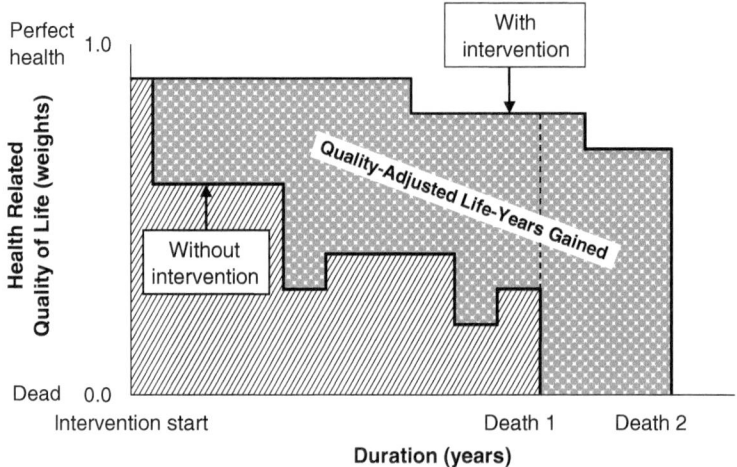

Fig. 6.2 Concept of QALY (Source: Drummond [3])

humanistic outcomes represent the provider perspective and the patient perspective, respectively [7].

Health-care utilizations involves hospitalizations, emergency department visits, clinic visits, and drug usages [21]. They are efficient and interpretable proxies for health-care costs, since health-care costs depend on numerous factors such as different reimbursement structures, volume discounts, and institutional overhead [7]. In addition, health-care utilizations may be generalizable to other health-care systems because they are not dependent on a reimbursement structure such as Medicare [7].

Costs include direct costs and indirect costs. The direct costs consist of medical costs and nonmedical costs. Medical costs indicate the costs for health-care utilizations, which may vary by institution or location [7]. The nonmedical costs indicate the additional costs associated with utilizing health-care services (e.g., nursing home, transportation to health-care provider, child daycare, and support from family).

Indirect costs consist of opportunity costs and externalities. Opportunity costs indicate the loss of productivity of patients due to the illness, including the costs for loss of life year (mortality), disability, absenteeism, presenteeism, and days missed from work. The costs for externalities indicate the productivity loss of other persons due to patients' illness, such as the costs for caretakers' inability to work.

There are three methods for estimating indirect costs: (1) the human capital method, (2) the friction cost method, and (3) the willingness-to-pay method. The human capital method estimates lost productivity in terms of lost earnings. The friction cost method estimates only the production loss during the replacement time of a worker (the friction period for hiring a new worker). The willingness-to-pay method estimates the amounts that people are willing to pay to reduce the probability of illness or death.

The human capital method is the most commonly used, and the willingness-to-pay method usually provides a higher estimate of the value of life than the human capital method [22]. The friction method is rarely used because estimating losses in the friction period requires extensive data [22].

Which costs should be included depends on the perspective of the study. Direct medical costs can be calculated from a health-care system perspective, while the indirect costs come from an employer perspective. From the societal perspective, direct and indirect costs to patients, employers, and payer should be considered.

Economic Evaluation Methods

Economic evaluation is a methodology used to evaluate an intervention in health care or to compare different strategies on the same target effectiveness. It is widely used in evaluating new drug products for pharmaceutical companies as well as new interventions in health care. The results of economic evaluation provide a basis for justifying an introduction of a new approach compared to the status quo or different approaches.

The economic evaluation is categorized into two methods, depending on the resources used, as shown in Fig. 6.3. The first category considers only costs to

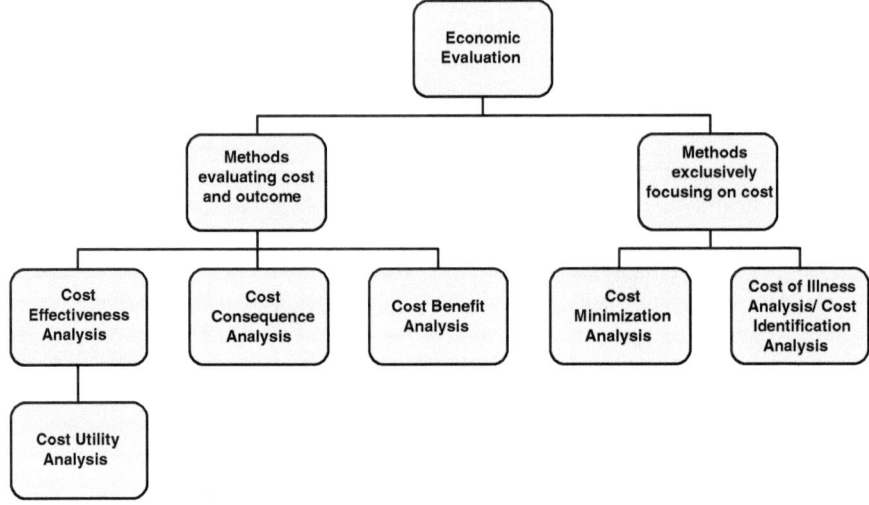

Fig. 6.3 Categories of economic evaluations

evaluate the intervention. It includes the cost-minimization analysis (CMA), the cost illness analysis (COI), and the cost-identification analysis (CIA). The second category takes into account costs and outcomes to evaluate the intervention allowing the different effectiveness on health outcomes. It includes the cost-effectiveness analysis (CEA), the cost-utility analysis (CUA), the cost-consequence analysis (CCA), and the cost-benefit analysis (CBA).

Cost-Effectiveness Analysis (CEA)

Introduction

The cost-effectiveness analysis (CEA) is the most common type of economic evaluation. It consists of costs and outcomes including non-monetary measures (natural units) of health outcomes. The CEA compares the costs and outcomes of alternative approaches to reaching the "same" objective. It aims to determine which alternative accomplishes a given objective at the least cost.

The CEA uses natural units such as years of life saved (YLS) and symptom-free days. Resources (costs) are valued in monetary units ($). Consequently, results are expressed as cost per natural units (e.g., $/YLS).

This approach has the following advantages. (1) It compares various forms of therapy (e.g., different classes of drugs to treat the same disease). (2) It is useful and acceptable for physicians and payers. (3) It allows evaluation of intermediate and short-term outcomes.

Methods

Conducting CEA consists of following steps: (1) designing the model or study, (2) collecting data on costs and benefits, (3) conducting a base-case analysis, and (4) solving an uncertainty.

Designing the Model or Study

The first step is to define the status quo (baseline case), which means the status in the absence of the intervention [23]. The cost and benefit without intervention will be baseline cost and benefit.

The second step is to define an intervention to be compared with the baseline case. One or more interventions may be compared with the baseline case. The intervention will add cost and benefit additional to those of the baseline case.

The third step is to define the perspectives of the study before collecting data on costs and benefits. The perspective may be payer, patient, hospital, health-care system, or society. Depending on the perspective, the categories to be considered in costs and benefits will differ. As the perspective becomes higher level, the costs and benefits to be considered will become larger.

Collecting Data of Cost and Benefit

The fourth step is to identify and categorize costs and benefits, which may include direct measures and indirect measures [23]. Direct costs include medical costs and intervention costs, while indirect costs include loss of productivity as well as medical costs of complications or adverse events. The benefits include health outcomes of patients considering adverse events.

Then, the costs need to be monetized in terms of a currency (e.g., US dollars), because currency units are generally understandable for people [23]. Also, the benefits of interest should be identified and quantified in terms of units of effectiveness. The benefits will be the effectiveness of intervention to measure the success of the intervention [23].

The fifth step is to specify a time frame for analysis. The time is typically measured in years, but researchers may use other units of time [23]. The time frame may be within or greater than 1 year. The time frame is directly related to discounting the costs and benefits of different years. That is, the costs and benefits should be discounted if the time frame is more than 1 year.

The reason for discounting costs and benefits of different years is that the values of benefits and costs in the current year differ from those in other years due to inflation rates, interest rates, or time preference. Namely, $1 in the current year does not have equal value to $1 in next year because $1 in the current year can generate interest (opportunity cost) over the course of a year or because the real value of $1 may decrease over time due to inflation. In addition, people prefer today's benefits to those of the future [23].

Actual discounting methods consist of two components: inflating past costs and discounting future costs and benefits. The past costs are inflated to current-year values using the consumer price index (CPI) [24]. Depending on the subject of analysis, a subcategory of CPI, such as medical care CPI, may be used to measure inflation. The future costs and benefits are discounted at specific annual rate (typically 3–5 %) to be converted to the present value. Past benefits are not inflated to current-year value because no reference method is available. However, if the past benefits are measured in monetary value ($), inflation should be applied.

For the conversion of currencies among different countries, the exchange rate or the purchasing power parity (PPP) is used to account for price differences across countries [3, 25]. Applying the PPP and exchange rate together is the best choice. If only one method should be chosen, the PPP is better choice than the exchange rate for conversion.

Conducting Base-Case Analysis

The base-case analysis is conducted to determine the incremental cost-effectiveness ratio (ICER) of intervention compared to the status quo [3]. An ICER indicates an additional amount paid to obtain an additional benefit using two components: an incremental cost (numerator) and an incremental effectiveness (denominator) [3].

$$ICER = \frac{Incremental\,Cost}{Incremental\,Effectiveness} = \frac{\left(Cost\,of\,Intervention - Cost\,of\,Baseline\right)}{\left(Effect\,of\,Intervention - Effect\,of\,Baseline\right)}$$

The results of analysis will be split into four categories in the incremental cost-effectiveness plane (Fig. 6.4) depending on values of ICER, incremental cost, and incremental effectiveness. A negative ICER indicates that an intervention (or baseline) is dominating the baseline (or intervention). The dominating strategy is strongly preferred over the dominated strategy because it has more effectiveness and less cost. For instance, if the intervention is more effective ($+\Delta E$) and less costly ($-\Delta C$) than the baseline, an ICER will be negative where the intervention is a dominant case. No further evaluation is required for the dominant cases.

A positive ICER is the main target to evaluate the cost-effectiveness of intervention, where the intervention is more (less) costly and more (less) effective than the baseline. The criterion for justifying the cost-effectiveness is whether the ICER is below the willingness-to-pay (WTP), which indicates the amount of monetary value willing to pay for obtaining an additional benefit. For instance, if an ICER is less than the WTP, the intervention is determined to be cost-effective compared to the baseline.

If two or more interventions are compared to the baseline, the smaller ICER is the better choice. The smaller ICER means that we may incur a smaller cost to obtain the same additional effect than with other choices.

However, if two or more interventions have the same ICERs, the evaluation is not available because ICER gives no idea of the size (or scale) of the intervention. Alternative measures are the net monetary benefit (NMB) and net health benefit (NHB) based on the WTP: $NMB = (WTP * \Delta E) - \Delta C$ and $NHB = \Delta E - (\Delta C / WTP)$. The greater is the better.

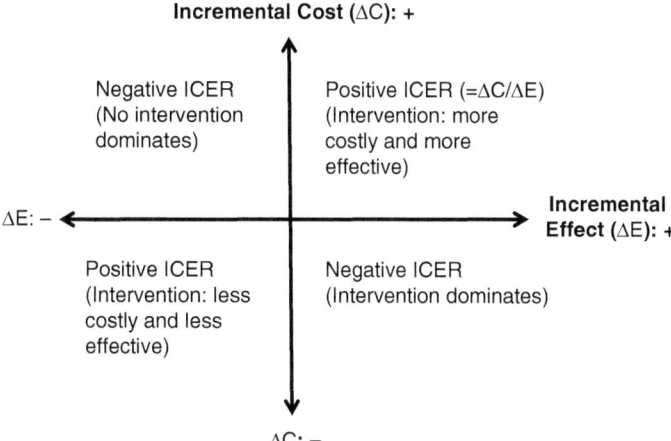

Incremental Cost (ΔC): +

Negative ICER
(No intervention
dominates)

Positive ICER (=ΔC/ΔE)
(Intervention: more
costly and more
effective)

ΔE: −

**Incremental
Effect (ΔE): +**

Positive ICER
(Intervention: less
costly and less
effective)

Negative ICER
(Intervention dominates)

ΔC: −

Fig. 6.4 Incremental cost-effectiveness plane (Source: Drummond [3])

Solving an Uncertainty

The weak point of base-case analysis is that the uncertainty in the model or study has not been solved. How to deal with uncertainties is depending on whether the study design is a clinical trial or a decision-analytic model. For a clinical trial study using patient-level data such as randomized controlled trial, a bootstrapping method is employed to obtain 95 % confidence interval of ICERs and then to create a cost-effectiveness acceptability curve [3, 26].

For a decision-analytic model, the most common uncertainty is that the values of parameters in the model may differ in circumstances with different assumptions. Two methods are employed: (1) a standard sensitivity analysis and (2) a probabilistic sensitivity analysis using Monte Carlo simulation. The standard sensitivity analysis sets the range of parameter values to test whether the result of base-case analysis changes on the range of parameter values (sensitive or not to the change of parameter value). It includes one-way or two-way sensitivity analysis depending on one or two parameters included for testing sensitivity, holding all else constant.

The probabilistic sensitivity analysis includes the uncertainty of all parameters, by assigning ranges and distributions to parameters and using Monte Carlo simulation. This analysis generates 95 % confidence interval of ICERs and then creates cost-effectiveness acceptability curve. It has the advantage that it can simultaneously deal with a large number of parameters and can indicate the degree of confidence [27].

Limitations

The limitation of CEA is that alternatives must have similar outcomes. For instance, we cannot compare cost/reduction in hemoglobin A1C with cost/reduction in systolic blood pressure.

Example Study

Kattan and colleagues (2005) conducted a randomized, controlled trial for an environmental intervention study of inner-city asthma in seven urban areas in the United States in 2001 [28]. The study objective was to determine the ICER of the environmental intervention compared to the status quo (no intervention). The target population was children, aged 5–11, with asthma. The time frame for intervention was 2 years. A 3 % discount rate was used to discount the second-year costs and benefits. The health outcome measured was the number of annual symptom-free days (SFD) per child. The total annual cost included the intervention cost (for the intervention group only) and the health service utilization costs. All costs were converted to 2001 US dollars. As a result, the incremental cost of intervention was $1,042, and the incremental benefit of intervention was 37.8 SFDs per child over the study period. Therefore, the ICER was $27.57 per additional SFD (95 % confidence interval: $7.46~$67.42). If a child is willing to pay $100 per additional SFD, the intervention is definitely cost-effective because the ICER is less than $100 of the willingness to pay (WTP).

Cost-Utility Analysis (CUA)

The cost-utility analysis (CUA) is defined as a form of CEA in which outcomes are adjusted for patient preferences (utility). The utility is the value placed on a level of health status measured by the preferences [29]. The most commonly used utility is the quality-adjusted life year (QALY), which combines benefits of survival and quality of life. CUA accounts for not only life span but also the quality of patients' lives by measuring patient utilities [11].

The CUA is most commonly used in order to allocate limited resources among interventions that have different objectives and benefits within the health-care sector [3]. That is, it determines the allocative efficiency of resources among interventions within the health-care sector only.

The CUA has the following characteristics. (1) The resources are measured in monetary units ($). (2) The consequences are measured in QALYs. (3) The results are reported as $/QALY such as average CU ratio and incremental CU ratio.

The first advantage of a CUA is that it makes different types of outcomes and disease comparable using QALY, which combines multiple outcomes into one unit [11]. The second advantage is that morbidity and mortality were incorporated into QALY [11]. The third advantage is that there is no need to monetize health outcomes [11].

The disadvantage of a CUA is that the value of QALY may be different depending on the methods used to estimate utilities [11]. The representative methods to estimate utilities are EQ-5D, Short Form 6D, Quality of Well-Being, and Health Utilities Index as shown in Table **6.1**. Those methods have different numbers of attributes and use different preference measurements to construct the health-related quality of life. Those differences result in the differences in values of QALY.

Table 6.1 Comparison of health-related quality of life measures

	Attributes	Preference measurement method
Quality of Well-Being	4	Category scaling
EQ-5D	5 (245 health states)	Time-Trade-Off
Short Form 6D	249 health states	Utility scaling
Health Utilities Index	7 (HUI2) 8 (HUI3)	Standard gambling and visual analogue scaling

Source: Drummond [3]

Methods

The methods to conduct CUA are almost the same as those of CEA. Therefore, all methods in CEA are applied in CUA. However, there are a few differences between CEA and CUA.

While CEA reports ICERs as cost per natural unit of effect, CUA reports ICERs as cost per QALY gained. While CEA may use intermediate outcomes for measuring effectiveness, CUA requires the final outcome because it is hard to link intermediate outcome and QALY [11]. In addition, the uncertainty related to the QALY measurement may critically impact the results of CUA. Therefore, sensitivity analysis is necessary to examine the results' robustness to the QALY changes [11].

Example Study

Briggs and colleagues (2010) conducted a cost-utility analysis of three treatment interventions for patients with COPD [30]. The interventions were the long-acting β_2-agonist salmeterol (Salm) 50 mg and the inhaled corticosteroid fluticasone propionate (FP) 500 mg, individually and as a fixed-dose combination (SFC), compared to the placebo (P) group. They conducted the randomized controlled trial for patients with COPD during 3 years in 42 countries. Data on health status and medical recourse use was collected. The health status was measured using the EQ-5D questionnaire in order to get the health-related quality of life (HRQL). A survival analysis was conducted to get the mortality data. Finally, the QALYs were obtained by combining the expected life year and the HRQL. The costs included hospitalizations, physician visits, therapy, medications, and productivity losses. All costs in foreign countries were converted to US dollars using the purchasing power parity. If needed, the costs were also inflated to 2007-year dollars. The ICERs among the three treatments, compared to the placebo group, were obtained for each country and pooled data. The pooled data showed ICERs of $43,600 (SFC), $197,000 (Salm), and $78,000 (FT) per QALY gained, compared to the P group. Therefore, SFC is determined to be most cost-effective, and Salm is to be least cost-effective. That is, SFC is preferred to other medications.

Cost-Consequence Analysis (CCA)

The cost-consequence analysis (CCA) is designed to calculate resources and outcomes without aggregating them into cost-outcome ratios [31]. It provides the most comprehensive presentation of information on costs and benefits [32].

It has the following characteristics. (1) Resources are measured in monetary units. (2) Outcomes are measured in multiple ways. (3) Results are presented in a tabular format.

Its advantages are transparency, flexibility, simplicity of concept, avoidance of controversies, and comprehensiveness. The disadvantage is that it does not indicate the relative importance of the different outcomes.

Methods

The methods to conduct CCA are almost same as those of CEA. Therefore, most methods in CEA are applied in CCA. However, there are a few differences between CEA and CCA.

The first is that CCA lists all relevant costs and outcomes consisting of the following components: (1) direct medical costs, (2) direct nonmedical costs, (3) indirect costs, (4) quality of life impacts, (5) utility impacts, and (6) clinical outcomes [32]. The second difference is that CCA does not provide any decision criterion because all information is disaggregated.

Example Study

Kroese and colleagues (2011) conducted a cost-consequence analysis of specialized rheumatology nurse (SRN) care compared to rheumatologist (RMT) care (usual care) in the diagnostic process for fibromyalgia (FM) in the Netherlands [33]. They conducted a 9-month randomized, controlled trial to measure costs and consequences for patients between the SRN group and the usual care group. The analysis was conducted from the health care and societal perspectives. The measured health outcomes included patients' satisfaction, HRQL, functional status, fatigue, self-efficacy, medical consumption, and social participation. The costs included health-care consumption, patient and family cost, and productivity costs using the cost diary method in terms of societal perspective. All costs were converted into 2007 prices using the Dutch consumer price index. Productivity losses were calculated using the human capital approach. Finally, the paper showed the consequences of costs and health outcomes in tabular formats between the SRN group and the usual care group.

Cost-Benefit Analysis (CBA)

The cost-benefit analysis (CBA) compares resources and outcomes of a program or treatment measured in monetary units. Its objectives are to identify the alternative with the greatest net benefit and to determine whether a good or service has positive net benefits.

The CBA can compare alternatives with similar and dissimilar outcomes. Resources and outcomes are measured in monetary units. Then, the results are reported as net benefit (B-C) and benefit-to-cost ratio (B/C).

This analysis has the following advantages. (1) It can compare widely varying programs and services with different outcomes. That is, CBA allows us to evaluate allocative efficiency among interventions between health care and other sectors. (2) It is easily understood: it is the only technique with a definitive, self-contained decision rule for evaluating a single intervention. That is, if the net benefit is positive, the intervention should be justified.

Methods

The methods to conduct CBA are similar to those of CEA. Therefore, most methods in CEA are applied in CBA. However, there were a few differences between CEA and CBA.

First of all, while CEA uses the natural unit of effectiveness, CBA needs to monetize benefits [23]. The benefits include non-market goods and services (e.g., saved caregivers' time), cost avoidance (e.g., reduced medical cost), saved time, and increased health outcomes (e.g., increased life years or QALY) [23].

The most controversial aspect of monetizing benefits is how to place a dollar value on benefits, for instance, if a year of life is saved (death averted), how to value a year of life in CBA. Two methods have been used in valuing a year of life: (1) the human capital approach and (2) the willingness-to-pay approach. The human capital approach estimates the present value of lifetime earnings that represents the productivity gains from extending life. The WTP approach estimates the amounts that people are willing to pay to reduce the probability of dying. The second approach can measure total value of life, including foregone earnings and the non-market value of life.

Secondly, with regard to the method to evaluate the intervention program, CBA determines the benefit-cost ratio (BCR=incremental benefit/incremental cost) and the net benefit amount (incremental benefit-incremental cost). The criteria are whether BCR>1 or B-C>0. If BCR>1, then acceptance of the intervention program is justified because a $1 investment resulted in a benefit greater than $1.

Limitations

CBA has the following limitations. (1) The valuation of outcomes in monetary units can be challenging. That is, valuing human life may be viewed as unethical. (2) It is not widely accepted in the health-care environment. (3) CBA depends on a model with significant assumptions. Therefore, its validation is necessary.

Example Study

Runge and colleagues (2006) conducted a cost-benefit analysis of a web-based patient education intervention compared to no intervention status among patients with asthma in Germany [34]. The study objective was to determine whether the internet-based education program (IEP), added to the standardized patient management program (SPMP), improves health outcomes of patients with asthma. The target patients were children and adolescents aged 8–16 years. The study period was 6 months in a nonrandomized trial. Two intervention groups had SPMP and one of them had IEP in addition to SPMP, compared to a control group without any education program. The costs included direct medical costs (medical care visits, emergency department visits, and inpatient care), direct nonmedical costs (transportation costs and internet access costs), and indirect costs (caregivers' loss of workdays due to a child's asthma). Intervention costs for SPMP and IEP were calculated also. The benefits were obtained by subtracting the costs between the control group and the intervention groups. Both intervention groups showed cost savings compared to the control group. Prices were adjusted to 2001-year values. There was no discounting, since the study period was within 1 year. The net benefit was calculated by subtracting the intervention costs from the benefits. The benefit-cost ratio was obtained as a ratio of benefits to intervention costs. The results showed that both intervention groups had decreased health-care utilizations. From a payer perspective, the benefit-cost ratio was 0.55 for SPMP group and 0.79 for SPMP + IEP group. For patients with moderate or severe asthma, the benefit-cost ratio was 1.07 for SPMP group and 1.42 for SPMP + IEP group. The interventions were justifiable for patients with moderate or severe asthma since the benefit-cost ratio was greater than 1. In addition, the intervention (SPMP + IEP) was better than the intervention (SPMP only) due to the higher benefit-cost ratio.

Cost-Minimization Analysis (CMA)

The cost-minimization analysis (CMA) is designed to compare the cost of two or more alternatives that have identical outcomes. Its objective is to identify the least expensive alternative, thereby minimizing cost.

This analysis has the following characteristics. (1) Alternatives are proven or assumed identical. (2) Resources are valued in monetary units ($). (3) Outcomes are identical and not valued. (4) Results are expressed in monetary units ($).

CMA is mostly useful for comparing branded versus generic efficacy (acquisition costs). It is often used for comparison of me-too drugs despite potential slight differences in effectiveness or adverse events. The other potential application is for the same drug in different formulations, considering acquisition cost and resource use.

Methods

The methods to conduct CMA are similar to those of CEA. Therefore, most methods in CEA are applied in CMA. However, there are a few differences between CEA and CMA.

The first difference is that CMA considers only costs with assumption of identical effectiveness. If the effectiveness of intervention is different from the original program, CMA is not applicable. That is, it has a limited application because normally the benefit with interventions differs from that without intervention.

The second difference is the method to evaluate the intervention program. The criterion is the minimum cost between the intervention and the original program. The program with the minimum cost is accepted.

Limitations

The limitation of CMA is that it is not applicable for innovations that offer additional outcome or fewer side effects.

Example Study

Dasta and colleagues (2010) conducted a cost-minimization analysis of dexmedetomidine compared to midazolam among mechanically ventilated patients in an intensive care unit (ICU) [35]. The randomized, controlled trial was conducted to determine the total ICU cost difference between patients with each medication by assuming that both medications have the identical effectiveness. Total ICU costs included cost of ICU stay, cost of mechanical ventilation, cost of treating adverse drug reaction, and cost of study medication. All costs were converted to 2007 US dollars using the medical care consumer price index. Results of primary analysis showed that the acquisition cost of dexmedetomidine ($1,166) was much higher than that of midazolam ($60). However, the dexmedetomidine group showed cost savings (median cost) of $9,679 compared to the midazolam group. The costs for ICU stay and mechanical ventilation were the main contributors (98.5 %) to the cost difference. Therefore, dexmedetomidine was preferred to midazolam due to the cost-saving result with identical effectiveness.

Cost-of-Illness Analysis (COI)/Cost-Identification Analysis (CIA)

The cost-of-illness study (COI) is designed to determine the total economic impact of a disease on society. It estimates the burden of a specific disease from different perspectives [36]. The perspectives can be state or government, employer, health insurance/sickness fund, or individual (patients, families, and others). On the whole, cost-identification studies determine the total cost burden of a treatment on a population [7].

COI has the following characteristics. (1) It identifies, measures, and values all direct and indirect costs. (2) It evaluates current status. (3) It does not address treatment efficacy.

Methods

The methods to conduct COI follow the steps below.

First, the perspective of the study should be determined. It may be the perspective of the health-care system, the employer, or the society. Depending on the perspective of study, the components of total cost may vary. For instance, for the health-care system perspective, the direct costs, including medical and nonmedical costs, are enough. For the employer perspective, the indirect costs (productivity loss) may be sufficient. For the societal perspective, all costs should be included.

The second step is to determine which type of cost will be estimated. Two types of cost can be estimated in COI: total costs and incremental costs [37]. Estimating total costs of a disease does not require a comparison group and uses the Sum_All Medical method or the Sum_Diagnosis Specific method [37]. The Sum_All Medical method identifies patients with a diagnosis of disease and sums all costs, while the Sum_Diagnosis Specific method identifies patients with a primary diagnosis of disease and sums costs for treating that diagnosis [37].

Estimating incremental costs requires a comparison group and uses the matched-control method or the regression method [37]. The matched-control method identifies all patients with a diagnosis, sums costs, and then calculates the difference in average costs between the case group and the matched-control group [37]. The regression method identifies all patients with a diagnosis, sums costs, and then conduces a regression analysis to obtain the estimated coefficient of case–control indicator that shows the incremental costs [37].

The third step is to estimate the annual total costs of disease, composed of direct costs and indirect costs. How to obtain the annual total costs has two approaches depending on how to use the epidemiological data [38]. The first one is the prevalence approach, which estimates the annual cost of illness based on one period (e.g., 1 year) regardless of the date of the onset of illness [22]. The second one is the incidence approach, which estimates the lifetime cost of illness from onset to conclusion within a study period (e.g., 1 year) [22]. The former approach is more common than the latter because the former requires less data and fewer assumptions than the latter [22].

The fourth step is to estimate direct costs, consisting of medical costs and non-medical costs. Estimating direct costs uses one of two methods [39]. The first method is top-down costing, which allocates national health-care expenditures to each disease category based on the primary diagnosis using International Classification of Diseases (ICD) code [39]. The second method is bottom-up costing, which estimates the quantity of health inputs used and the unit costs of the inputs and then multiplies the unit costs by the quantities [39]. Bottom-up costing requires much greater input data at a detailed level than top-down costing [39].

Generally, the incidence approach employs the bottom-up costing method to obtain the lifetime costs of illness [39]. On the whole, the prevalence approach employs the top-down costing method to assign portions of a revealed total expenditure to each category of a broad disease [39].

The fifth step is to estimate indirect costs, if necessary, depending on the perspective of the study. Indirect costs are estimated using one of three methods: (1) the human capital method, (2) the friction cost method, and (3) the willingness-to-pay method.

The sixth step is to inflate the past-year value to a same-year value and to discount the future-year value to a same-year value.

Limitations

COI has the following limitations. (1) It is useful only for status analysis. It is not useful for resource prioritization or making decisions [40]. (2) It may have large percentage of indirect cost, which can vary considerably depending on the methodology used (human capital vs. friction cost). (3) It does not compare treatment alternatives [40].

Example Study

Stock and colleagues (2005) conducted a cost-of-illness analysis on asthma in order to estimate the cost burden of asthma in Germany [41]. The analysis examined claims data and national statistics to get cost data, based on the societal perspective, in 1999. The total costs included direct costs and indirect costs. Direct costs included the following categories: inpatient care, outpatient care, and inpatient rehabilitation. Indirect costs included sick benefit, early retirement, and premature death. For early retirement and premature death, the productivity loss was calculated using the human capital approach. The results showed that the total direct costs for treating asthma were €690.4 million (hospital costs, €48.2 million; inpatient rehabilitation, €62.5 million; medication costs, €579.7 million). The total productivity losses were €2.05 billion (sick benefit, €1194.8 million; early retirement, €610.2 million; premature death, €244.5 million). Total costs for asthma amounted to €2.74 billion, including direct costs and indirect costs. The indirect costs made up 74.8 % of total costs.

References

1. Porter ME (2010) What is value in health care? N Engl J Med 363(26):2477–2481
2. Samuelson PA, Nordhaus WD (2010) Economics, vol xxiv, 19th edn, The McGraw-Hill series economics. McGraw-Hill Irwin, Boston, p 715
3. Drummond M (2005) Methods for the economic evaluation of health care programmes, 3rd edn, Oxford medical publications. Oxford University Press, Oxford, New York, p 379
4. Motheral B (1997) Outcomes management: the why, what, and how of data collection. J Manag Care Pharm 3:345–351
5. Kozma CM, Reeder CE, Schulz RM (1993) Economic, clinical, and humanistic outcomes: a planning model for pharmacoeconomic research. Clin Ther 15(6):1121–1132; discussion 1120
6. Gunter MJ (1999) The role of the ECHO model in outcomes research and clinical practice improvement. Am J Manag Care 5(4 Suppl):S217–S224
7. Priscilla Velentgas P et al (eds) (2013) Developing a protocol for observational comparative effectiveness research: a user's guide. Agency for Healthcare Research and Quality (US), Rockville
8. Herman CR et al (2013) Development of a predictive model for major adverse cardiac events in a coronary artery bypass and valve population. J Cardiothorac Surg 8(1):177
9. U.S. Department of Health and Human Services. Office of Disease Prevention and Health Promotion, Healthy People 2020; Health-Related Quality of Life and Well-Being, Washington, DC
10. Guyatt GH, Feeny DH, Patrick DL (1993) Measuring health-related quality of life. Ann Intern Med 118(8):622–629
11. MacKinnon GE (2011) Understanding health outcomes and pharmacoeconomics. Jones and Bartlett Publishers, Burlington, MA
12. U.S. Department of Health and Human Services, Food and Drug Administration (2009) Guidance for industry: patient-reported outcome measures: use in medical product development to support labeling claims. Available at http://www.fda.gov/downloads/Drugs/GuidanceComplianceRegulatoryInformation/Guidances/UCM193282.pdf
13. Stamuli E (2011) Health outcomes in economic evaluation: who should value health? Br Med Bull 97:197–210
14. Torrance GW (1986) Measurement of health state utilities for economic appraisal. J Health Econ 5(1):1–30
15. Torrance GW (1987) Utility approach to measuring health-related quality of life. J Chronic Dis 40(6):593–603
16. Feeny D et al (1995) Multi-attribute health status classification systems. Health Utilities Index. Pharmacoeconomics 7(6):490–502
17. Feeny D et al (2004) Comparing directly measured standard gamble scores to HUI2 and HUI3 utility scores: group- and individual-level comparisons. Soc Sci Med 58(4):799–809
18. The EuroQol Group (1990) EuroQol—a new facility for the measurement of health-related quality of life. Health Policy 16(3):199–208
19. Brazier J et al (2008) Estimation of a preference-based index from a condition-specific measure: the King's Health Questionnaire. Med Decis Making 28(1):113–126
20. Lenert L, Kaplan RM (2000) Validity and interpretation of preference-based measures of health-related quality of life. Med Care 38(9 Suppl):II138–II150
21. Cheng Y et al (2013) Economic, clinical, and humanistic outcomes (ECHOs) of pharmaceutical care services for minority patients: a literature review. Res Social Adm Pharm 9(3): 311–329
22. Segel JE (2006) Cost-of-illness studies—A primer. RTI-UNC Center of Excellence in Health Promotion Economics, pp 1–39
23. Cellini SR, Kee JE (2010) Cost-effectiveness and cost-benefit analysis. Handbook of practical program evaluation. Jossey-Bass, San Francisco, CA, p 493

24. Consumer price index- all urban consumers (2014) [cited 17 Dec 2014]. Available from: http://www.bls.gov/data
25. OECD. StatExtracts. Purchasing Power Parities (PPP) Statistics (2014) [cited 17 Dec 2014]. Available from: http://stats.oecd.org/
26. Ramsey SD, Willke RJ, Glick H, et al (2015) Cost-effectiveness analysis alongside clinical trials II-An ISPOR Good Research Practices Task Force report. Value in health : the journal of the International Society for Pharmacoeconomics and Outcomes Research 18(2):161–172
27. Robinson R (1993) Economic evaluation and health care. What does it mean? BMJ 307(6905):670–673
28. Kattan M et al (2005) Cost-effectiveness of a home-based environmental intervention for inner-city children with asthma. J Allergy Clin Immunol 116(5):1058–1063
29. Bootman JL, Townsend RJ, McGhan WF (2005) Principles of pharmacoeconomics, vol x, 3rd edn. Harvey Whitney Books Co, Cincinnati, p 409
30. Briggs AH et al (2010) Is treatment with ICS and LABA cost-effective for COPD? Multinational economic analysis of the TORCH study. Eur Respir J 35(3):532–539
31. Russell LB et al (1996) The role of cost-effectiveness analysis in health and medicine. JAMA 276(14):1172–1177
32. Mauskopf JA et al (1998) The role of cost-consequence analysis in healthcare decision-making. Pharmacoeconomics 13(3):277–288
33. Kroese ME et al (2011) Specialized rheumatology nurse substitutes for rheumatologists in the diagnostic process of fibromyalgia: a cost-consequence analysis and a randomized controlled trial. J Rheumatol 38(7):1413–1422
34. Runge C et al (2006) Outcomes of a web-based patient education program for asthmatic children and adolescents. Chest 129(3):581–593
35. Dasta JF et al (2010) A cost-minimization analysis of dexmedetomidine compared with midazolam for long-term sedation in the intensive care unit. Crit Care Med 38(2):497–503
36. Koopmanschap MA (1998) Cost-of-illness studies. Useful for health policy? Pharmacoeconomics 14(2):143–148
37. Akobundu E et al (2006) Cost-of-illness studies : a review of current methods. Pharmacoeconomics 24(9):869–890
38. Byford S, Torgerson DJ, Raftery J (2000) Economic note: cost of illness studies. BMJ 320(7245):1335
39. Tarricone R (2006) Cost-of-illness analysis: what room in health economics? Health Policy 77(1):51–63
40. Shiell A, Gerard K, Donaldson C (1987) Cost of illness studies: an aid to decision-making? Health Policy 8(3):317–323
41. Stock S et al (2005) Asthma: prevalence and cost of illness. Eur Respir J 25(1):47–53

Chapter 7
Medical Decision Making: When Evidence and Medical Culture Clash

Andy Bland and Bonnie Paris

Abstract A clinical practice guideline (CPG) is a recommendation for standardized workflow and decision -making for a specific clinical situation. Thousands of clinical practice guidelines exist, and the quality of guidelines varies. In Chap. 7, we examine why physicians do not follow agreed-upon evidence-based clinical practice guidelines. We discuss the problems and benefits of using clinical practice guidelines and how they are adopted into practice, providing examples of clinical practice guidelines for hand hygiene and perioperative beta blockers. We discuss the measurement of adherence to clinical practice guidelines and the effect of multiple medical conditions and multiple clinical guidelines on adherence. We discuss the disadvantages of applying individual behavior models to understand clinical practice guideline adoption and present several systems frameworks to aid in implementing clinical practice guidelines. Clinical practice guidelines will remain ubiquitous in modern medicine, and the quality of CPGs will improve over time. However, current information available online is not sufficient to support busy practitioners in decision making. A systems framework should be used to understand CPG adoption, and care should be taken in using CPG adherence as a performance metric.

There is a need for "decision-support systems that integrate clinical data with current, evidence-based, best-practice information and that provide information on when and why it may be appropriate to deviate from best practices" (Haynes (2005)

A. Bland, MD (✉)
Department of Medicine, HSHS Medical Group, Springfield, IL, USA

Department of Internal Medicine, University of Illinois College of Medicine at Peoria, Peoria, IL, USA

Hospital & Health Care, Springfield, IL, USA
e-mail: Andrew.Bland@hshs.org

B. Paris, PhD
Center for Outcomes Research, Department of Internal Medicine, University of Illinois College of Medicine at Peoria, Peoria, IL, USA
e-mail: blparis@uic.edu

© Springer International Publishing Switzerland 2016   83
C. Asche (ed.), *Applying Comparative Effectiveness Data to Medical Decision Making: A Practical Guide*, DOI 10.1007/978-3-319-23329-1_7

Evidence-based medicine. In: Building a better delivery system: a new engineering/ health care partnership. The National Academies Press, Washington, DC, pp 117– 118). Such a system would provide a relevant synthesis of EBM recommendations, potentially dangerous drug-drug interactions, and contradictory recommendations. This custom "patient- centered" clinical practice guideline could be incorporated into the electronic health record, and this would become the quality measurement standard by which the clinical care would be measured. This would avoid the dangerous paradox created by following clinical guidelines where good clinicians are punished for applying physiology, pathophysiology, pharmacology, and EBM to individual patients.

Thousands of clinical practice guidelines exist, and there are more than a dozen systems for evaluating the strength of evidence for recommendations. Different guidelines can offer conflicting recommendations, and the quality of guidelines varies [1]. In this chapter, we examine why physicians do not follow agreed-upon evidence-based clinical practice guidelines. We discuss the problems and benefits of using clinical practice guidelines and how they are adopted into practice. We discuss the measurement of adherence to clinical practice guidelines and the effect of multiple medical conditions and multiple clinical guidelines on adherence. We discuss the disadvantages of applying individual behavior models to understand clinical practice guideline adoption and present several systems frameworks to aid in implementing clinical practice guidelines.

Clinical practice guidelines are ubiquitous in modern medicine.

What Are Clinical Practice Guidelines?

A clinical practice guideline (CPG) is a recommendation for standardized workflow and decision making for a specific clinical situation. The recommendations included in a clinical practice guideline are "intended to optimize patient care" and "informed by a systematic review of evidence and an assessment of the benefits and harms of alternative care options" [1]. Figure 7.1 depicts the basic process by which evidence is transformed into a clinical practice guideline. However, the reality of guideline development is far more complex.

Who Creates CPGs?

CPGs are created by government organizations (e.g., CDC, NIH, VA), clinical specialty organizations (e.g., ACP, AMA), disease-specific organizations (e.g., AHA, AGA), and international organizations [1].

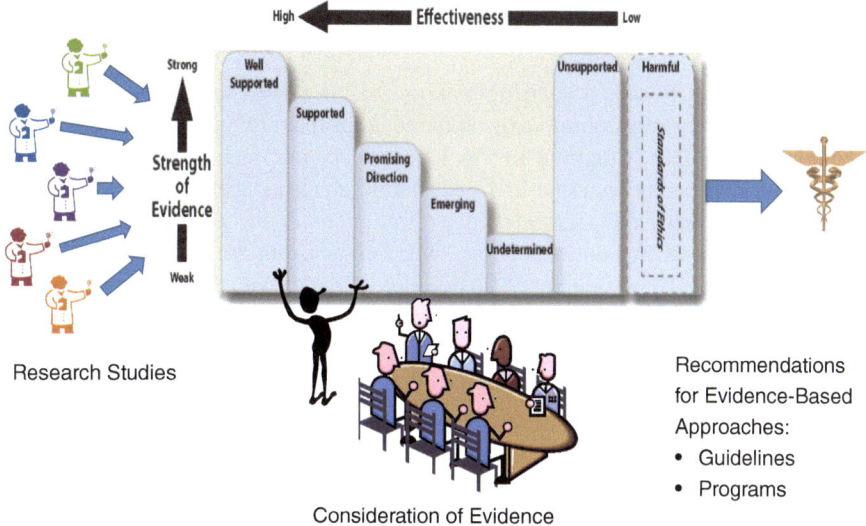

Fig. 7.1 How clinical practice guidelines are developed

Where Do You Find CPGs?

The National Guideline Clearinghouse (http://www.guideline.gov) is the main source for clinical practice guidelines in the United Sates. Currently, there are 103,529 citations on PubMed referencing the 2,603 currently active clinical practice guidelines. However, guideline documents can be lengthy, and multiple guidelines can exist concerning the same clinical situation. To alleviate these issues, the Journal of the American Medical Association has introduced a new series of "Clinical Guidelines Synopsis" articles to "concisely summarize guideline recommendations in a format designed for busy physicians" [2].

How Are CPGs Developed?

New guidelines are introduced and existing guidelines are modified on a continual basis, to keep current with what is known from research. Ideally, development of a clinical practice guideline would involve "a knowledgeable, multidisciplinary panel of experts and representatives from key affected groups" in a "methodologically rigorous, transparent, evidence-based" process to produce a single trustworthy guideline [1]. With more than a dozen systems for evaluating the strength of evidence from research studies and no central body responsible for guideline development, it is not surprising that multiple, sometimes conflicting guidelines exist concerning the same clinical situation.

How Are CPGs Used?

Caregivers use CPGs as a decision-making aid for a specific clinical situation. A CPG includes "strong, definitive recommendations that often warrant uniformity of practice" in the few "situations in which confidence in effect estimates is high and the balance between desirable and undesirable consequences is clear" [3]. More often, a trustworthy CPG acknowledges limitations of the current research base, uncertainty of expected outcomes, and "whether decisions are value and preference dependent" [3]. CPGs support but do not replace the provider's active role in clinical decision making [4], and using a CPG in practice can be fraught with challenges, even for a single patient and single guideline. Clinicians must apply the CPG recommendations considering the patient's other medical conditions, values, and preferences [5].

Administrators, quality officers, insurance plans, and those responsible for measuring successful practice find CPGs useful for generating metrics and care guides designed to reduce unnecessary variability and measure quality by creating a peer-reviewed, standard approach to clinical practice. For example, "adherence" to CPGs has been advocated as a quality metric in pay for performance for physicians. Care should be taken when using CPG adherence as a quality metric or a performance metric; the methods by which adherence to CPGs and attribution to care providers are determined should be agreed upon and a fair representation of care provider responsibility.

As discussed in the following section, the difficulty of applying CPGs is amplified when a patient has multiple medical conditions to which multiple CPGs apply.

What Are the Problems with Using CPGs?

Sometimes clinical guidelines are disputed, and sometimes they are wrong [6]. There are limits to our current knowledge of what the "right" answer is, whether it regards diagnosis or treatment. When there is insufficient evidence to support a "best practice" clinical guideline, multiple, sometimes conflicting guidelines exist, and recommendations can change over time when new evidence is taken into consideration. We discuss the effect of multiple medical conditions and multiple clinical guidelines on adherence. The use of CPGs in "real-life" patient situations where multiple CPGs, contradictory medications, and significant drug interactions exist presents another challenge to the appropriate use of CPGs in clinical practice.

With the aging of the population, the number of patients with multiple comorbid conditions continues to grow. In 1999, 48 % of Medicare-aged patients had three or more chronic conditions [7]. By 2012, that number had risen to 66 % [8]. Clinical practice guidelines are often developed by specialty societies focused on one disease state [7]. These guidelines are often developed from randomized controlled trials (RCTs) designed to isolate one study condition and exclude confounding variables.

Boyd and colleagues applied the appropriate CPGs to a hypothetical 79-year-old female with osteoporosis, osteoarthritis, type 2 diabetes, hypertension, and COPD [7]. Using the CPGs, they drafted a treatment plan involving seven different medications taken at five different times during the day. This exercise highlighted the difficulties in integrating recommendations from multiple CPGs: the medication recommended for treatment of hypertension (hydrochlorothiazide or HCTZ) can cause hyperglycemia and is contraindicated for a patient with diabetes, and multiple clinically relevant medication interactions were not addressed. For example, combining ASA and NSAIDS increases the risk of bleeding, and effectiveness of antihypertensives is decreased when combined with NSAIDS. The risk of acute kidney injury that comes with using ACE-I, diuretics, and NSAIDS together is not discussed in any practice guideline. The CPGs laboratory monitoring recommendations did not adequately address risk of drug interactions and how to monitor for adverse reactions.

The authors then abstracted the list of behavioral modifications required for the 79-year-old female and the clinician tasks required. The patient regimen required taking various medications at five specified times throughout the day and maintaining a strict diet that included monitoring the intake of sodium, potassium, saturated fat, cholesterol, magnesium, and calcium [7]. The patient would also need to check blood sugar daily, check her feet daily, and sit upright for 30 min on the day when alendronate was taken [7]. This represents an overwhelming number of tasks and amount of education to be completed by the physician and patient in a 15-min office visit. The sheer complexity of these tasks would require multiple visits, follow-up phone calls, check-ins, and reminders to accomplish.

The reality is that a multidisciplinary care team, the patient, and the patient's family will all be involved in chronic disease management. However, "most clinical practice guidelines generally focus on physician actions and patient behaviors and tend to underplay the potential contributions of other healthcare providers" [9] or informal caregivers. This example demonstrates some of the practical difficulties of applying CPGs to a population of patients with multiple conditions [10].

What Are the Benefits of Using CPGs?

CPGs hold the promise of improving quality of care [11] and supporting care providers and patients in making decisions informed by the best available research evidence [6, 11]. Use of evidence-based CPGs has been shown to improve the process of care, but more research is needed on the impact of CPG use on clinical outcomes [12].

One of the most successful collections of CPGs developed is the American Academy of Pediatrics "Red Book." First issued in 1938, this collection of CPGs addresses infectious disease practice guidelines ranging from routine immunizations to Ebola screening and treatment [13]. The Red Book is a ubiquitous resource in ambulatory clinics and is used for immunization guidance as a definitive source for vaccination initiation and catch-up [13].

In our residency clinic, one of our attending physicians is famous for answering any immunization question with "What did the Red Book say?" The trustworthiness and adoption of these CPGs is the gold standard that any CPG should aspire to.

How Are CPGs Adopted?

A clinical practice guideline is an innovation in the process of care. Factors affecting adoption of the innovation include characteristics of the innovation itself, communication channels, time, and the social system [14]. There are many interacting factors that determine the speed and success of clinical practice guideline adoption; Greenhalgh and colleagues [15] conducted a systematic review of literature and developed a unifying conceptual model of innovation in health service delivery and organization. The conceptual model was created "as a memory aide for considering the different aspects of a complex situation and their many interactions" [15]. Indeed, the conceptual model developed by Greenhalgh et al. is a comprehensive framework for understanding health service delivery innovations from a systems perspective.

In a case where there is compelling evidence supporting an approach as superior to other approaches and where a trustworthy guideline has been developed, that guideline may be considered a "gold standard" or "best practice." We can understand why a clinical practice guideline is not followed when the recommendations are contested or when there is weak evidence for the recommendations. *However, in cases where there is a "gold standard," why is a clinical practice guideline not followed?* Beyond unintended errors and sabotage [16], sometimes a CPG is not followed because there is a poor fit between the recommended actions and the work system.

Modern medicine is practiced in an interdisciplinary healthcare system, where physicians maintain primary responsibility for diagnosing and directing the care of patients [17]. In recognition of the tension between provider professionalism and healthcare systems structure [18], a research model for clinical practice guideline adoption should examine the users of the guideline, separately and in relation to the social system [1, 19, 20]. Successful adoption of CPGs into current practice also requires integrating the CPG into the existing electronic medical record [4, 21]. Holden and Karsh developed a multilevel model of health information technology behavior, based on sociotechnical systems and macroergonomics theory [22], that can be useful in understanding the adoption of CPGs.

Systems factors can influence behavior positively (e.g., when the "right" behavior is the "easy" behavior) or negatively (e.g., when a poor fit between the work system and the situation makes the "right" behavior impractical or impossible). Other common system issues are incentives that are not aligned with the desired behavior and a lack of timely, relevant performance feedback. Another way to conceptualize the relationships in the healthcare system relevant to CPG adoption is to use the Systems Engineering Initiative for Patient Safety 2.0 model, which incorporates the work systems model with Donabedian's healthcare structure-process-outcome model [23]. This model can be used to understand elements of the system and how they interact.

In this section, we describe several systems frameworks for understanding the adoption of any given clinical practice guideline. Current medical literature on CPG adoption relies on individual-based frameworks such as the stages of change model or the theory of planned behavior, but these frameworks focus on physician behavior only and do not adequately capture the other people and components of the system or of the interaction between the people and components. A recent IOM report stated that:

> The old underlying assumptions about what it means to be a physician—which continue to be reinforced in training—are in conflict with what is needed to provide care that is aligned with the six aims of the chasm report as well as foster a learning health system [24].

Until CPG adoption is understood from a systems perspective, there will continue to be failed implementation of "gold standard" clinical practice guidelines.

What Are Some Examples of CPG Adoption?

For readers who are new to systems science and research on dissemination and implementation, it may help to consider a historical example of clinical practice guideline adoption: hand hygiene. We then discuss adoption of guidelines for perioperative beta blockers.

Hand Hygiene

In 1847, Ignaz Semmelweis introduced the innovation of disinfecting providers' hands using a chlorine-based solution in an obstetrics ward in Vienna [25]. Hand hygiene practices are simple, effective, and inexpensive innovations that have been proven to save lives and reduce costs. Although hand hygiene practices have been widely adopted, *compliance* remains an area for improvement [25–27]. It is more accurate to view today's hand hygiene practices as a series of innovations adopted over time, with less effective methods discontinued and replaced by new innovations. We no longer use the chlorine-based solution introduced by Semmelweis, and our standards for when to perform hand hygiene have changed as well (e.g., any time a potential contamination occurs, not just between patients or after touching cadavers).

The story of Semmelweis highlights the importance of the social system in guideline adoption. Although now recognized as a pioneer of hand hygiene and hospital epidemiology [25], Semmelweis could not gain acceptance by his colleagues during his lifetime [28]. Put plainly, "Semmelweis was a genius, but he was also a lunatic, and that made him a failed genius" [26]. Semmelweis died in a public insane asylum just a few years after publishing his findings [28] and nearly 20 years passed before the innovation he championed began to gain recognition and acceptance [25, 28]. Semmelweis failed to account for the social system in which he worked, and he did not recognize his innovation as a threat to the medical culture of the time.

Hand hygiene remains a contemporary problem, with facility design (e.g., availability of sinks and hand sanitizer) [29, 30] and social factors (e.g., observed coworker behavior) [9, 30] playing important roles in compliance. Different theoretical perspectives can be used to understand the difficulties in improving hand hygiene compliance, with factors at the individual, team, and organizational levels [27]. Examining the different compliance rates for hand hygiene and different contexts of care in an operating room and a general inpatient unit highlights many of these factors [9].

Perioperative Beta Blockers

In the late 1990s, the evidence-based medicine (EBM) movement was sweeping across academic institutions. Propelled by the DCCT trial in the early 1990s, EBM was viewed as the tool to drive clinical decision making away from the "see one, do one, teach one" anecdotal medicine of the past century. The first edition of AHRQ's Making Health Care Safer white paper [31] trumpeted the use of beta blockers preoperatively as Number 2 on a list of 11 Clear Opportunities for Safety Improvement. It stated:

> The use of beta blockers to reduce perioperative cardiac events and mortality represents a major advance in perioperative medicine for some patients at intermediate and high risk for cardiac events during non-cardiac surgery. Wider use of this therapy should be promoted and studied, with future research focused on fine-tuning dosages and schedules and identifying populations of patients in which its use is cost-effective [31].

The AHRQ white paper acknowledges the lack of conclusive evidence: "Results from several well-designed clinical trials suggest that use of beta blockers in the perioperative period is associated with significant reductions in patient cardiac morbidity and mortality. In the future such therapy may reduce the need for additional tests and revascularization procedures, further reducing costs of care. However, several questions regarding its use remain, and should be topics of future research" [31]. The jump from this statement to the conclusion suggests a gap in the evidence that had not yet been plugged.

Neuman and colleagues provide a comprehensive history of CPGs for perioperative use of beta blockers and present a powerful figure tracking the total number of patients studied by year with an overlay of when each new recommendation regarding the use of beta blockers was released [32]. Of note: all of the strong positive practice guidelines were released from 1997 to 2002, when the total N was well below 2000. In 2006, when the N began to dramatically rise, dramatically revised statements designed to reduce the scope and effect of beta blockers dramatically increased, leading to a comment in the 2013 AHRQ Making Health Care Safer II report:

> Evidence that has emerged since the 2001 publication of 'Making Health Care Safer' indicates that perioperative beta blockers have mixed benefits and harms and should not be considered a patient safety practice for all patients [33].

In retrospect, it is easy to see why a provider may have resisted adopting the earlier guidelines, not believing the recommendations:

- Guidelines were based on two studies (expert opinion).
- They did not discuss or illustrate the complications many were seeing (evidence-common sense mismatch, comorbidities not addressed).
- Outcomes were not observed (does not apply to typical patient).
- There was conflicting evidence in the literature (conflicting guidelines).

The history of perioperative beta blocker CPGs "shows how the prestige that medical researchers and clinicians afford to randomized controlled trials can obscure important uncertainties surrounding new treatments, particularly when placed in political contexts that prioritize the rapid translation of research into practice" [32]. RCTs are important, but they are not appropriate for all research questions [34]. Physiology and study results are necessary, but not sufficient, to predict success of a guideline's recommended intervention. A sufficient number of patients should be studied before generating a clinical guideline for dissemination. In the meantime, conflicting data, observations, and opinions must be addressed in a transparent manner [35]. Focused analysis of large data sets could augment the RCT trial process by modeling the real-world observations that providers experience. This also allows a risk-benefit assessment, based on large data sets, that will help guideline creators assess potential risks and conflicts.

What Are the Barriers to CPG Adoption?

Cabana and colleagues conducted a systematic literature review to identify barriers to CPG adherence and organized their findings in a framework related to physician knowledge, attitudes, and behavior [36]. A qualitative study demonstrated the relevance of their framework, as all of the key factors identified by Cabana and colleagues were perceived as important barriers to CPG use by general practitioners [37]. Individual provider use of CPG can be influenced by provider factors such as personal differences in risk tolerance, the role of emotions in decision making, the role of self-perception and self-identity, and so on. These barriers are summarized by provider factors, patient factors, guideline factors, and organizational factors in

Table 7.1. The barriers identified indicate poor fit between the CPG and the work system. It is interesting that, although the framework used by Cabana and colleagues was focused on physician behavior, other systems factors were identified as barriers to CPG adoption [36].

Although the barriers to physician adherence to CPGs presented by Cabana and colleagues are a good starting point, their framework relies on individual behavior change theories [38, 39]. Physicians are no longer "lone wolf" practitioners working in a cottage industry; the practice of modern medicine is in the context of the healthcare system. It is important to consider the context in which the CPG is being used. Rather than bewailing provider "resistance to change," we should recognize that resisting adoption of a bad CPG is a correct choice [21]. In fact, there is some evidence that experts are less likely to adhere to a CPG when there are relevant patient-related factors that would "provide a reasonable basis for not following the CPG" [5]. Systems behavior models reflect the reality of this complexity, whereas individual behavior models do not include the important interaction between physician and patient.

What Are the Facilitators to CPG Adoption?

A recent international mixed methods study identified enabling factors for healthcare innovation such as CPGs [40]:

Table 7.1 Barriers to CPG adoption

Factor type	Factor description
Provider factors	Lack of familiarity
	Disagreement with evidence
	Lack of applicability
	Loss of autonomy
	Lack of outcome expectancy
	Lack of motivation
Patient factors	Patient preference contradicts
	Patient without ability to follow guideline
Guideline factors	Ambiguous guideline
	Conflicting guidelines
	Comorbidity not addressed
	Does not apply to typical patient
	Out of date
	Ambiguous
	Too complex
	Evidence-"common sense" mismatch
Organizational factors	Lack of time
	Lack of resources
	System constraints
	Misaligned financial incentives

Adapted from Cabana et al. [36]

- Standards and protocols
- Communication channels across and beyond health care
- Transparency of findings and data demonstrating success
- Funding for research, development, and diffusion
- Specific resource to identify and promote innovation
- IT and informatics
- Vision and strategy
- Incentives and rewards

The authors emphasized the importance of understanding broader context and system characteristics, and they identified seven factors "of essential cultural dynamics, which are the behaviors, beliefs, and practices of healthcare organizations and their workforces" [40]. The seven essential factors are:

- Empowering patients
- Engaging healthcare professionals
- Adapting innovations to the local context
- Identifying and supporting champions
- Promoting learning and new ways of working
- Eliminating legacy practices
- Promoting future transformation

The systems behavior models previously introduced can be used to understand the various facilitators and the interactions between system components that produce a "good fit" of the CPG and the work system.

Conclusions and Recommendations

Clinical practice guidelines will remain ubiquitous in modern medicine, and the quality of CPGs will improve over time [1]. Use of clinical practice guidelines, care pathways, and best practice guides is strongly advocated on the AHRQ website, where providers can review the known universe of clinical guidelines in a guideline matrix. Although the website allows several guidelines to be compared side by side, the information produced is not sufficient to support busy practitioners in decision making. A systems framework should be used to understand CPG adoption, and care should be taken in using CPG adherence as a performance metric.

There is a need for "decision-support systems that integrate clinical data with current, evidence-based, best-practice information and that provide information on when and why it may be appropriate to deviate from best practices" [4]. Such a system would provide a relevant synthesis of EBM recommendations, potentially dangerous drug interactions, and contradictory recommendations. This custom "patient-centered" clinical practice guideline could be incorporated into the electronic health record, and this would become the quality measurement standard by which clinical care would be measured. This would avoid the dangerous paradox that following clinical guidelines may create, where good clinicians are punished for applying physiology, pathophysiology, pharmacology, and EBM to individual patients.

References

1. IOM (Institute of Medicine) (2011) Clinical practice guidelines we can trust. Washington, DC: The National Academies Press.
2. Cifu AS, Davis AM, Livingston EH (2014) Introducing jama clinical guidelines synopsis. JAMA 312(12):1208–1209
3. Djulbegovic B, Guyatt GH (2014) Evidence-based practice is not synonymous with delivery of uniform health care. JAMA 312(13):1293–1294
4. Haynes B (2005) Evidence-based medicine. In: Building a better delivery system: a new engineering/health care partnership. The National Academies Press, Washington, DC, pp 117–118
5. Mercuri M, Sherbino J, Sedran RJ, Frank JR, Gafni A, Norman G (2015) When guidelines don't guide: the effect of patient context on management decisions based on clinical practice guidelines. Acad Med 90:191–196
6. Sox HC (2014) Do clinical guidelines still make sense? Yes. Ann Fam Med 12(3):200–201
7. Boyd CM, Darer J, Boult C, Fried LP, Boult L, Wu AW (2005) Clinical practice guidelines and quality of care for older patients with multiple comorbid diseases: implications for pay for performance. JAMA 294(6):716–724
8. Centers for Medicare and Medicaid Services (2012) Chronic conditions among Medicare Beneficiaries, Chartbook, 2012 Edition
9. McDonnell Norms Group (2006) Enhancing the use of clinical guidelines: a social norms perspective. J Am Coll Surg 202(5):826–836
10. Upshur RE (2014) Do clinical guidelines still make sense? No. Ann Fam Med 12(3):202–203
11. Woolf SH, Grol R, Hutchinson A, Eccles M, Grimshaw J (1999) Clinical guidelines: potential benefits, limitations, and harms of clinical guidelines. BMJ 318(7182):527–530
12. Lugtenberg M, Burgers JS, Westert GP (2009) Effects of evidence-based clinical practice guidelines on quality of care: a systematic review. Qual Saf Health Care 18(5):385–392
13. Pickering LK, Peter G, Shulman ST (2013) The red book through the ages. Pediatrics 132(5):898–906
14. Rogers EM (2003) Diffusion of innovations, 5th edn. Free Press, New York
15. Greenhalgh T, Robert G, Macfarlane F, Bate P, Kyriakidou O (2004) Diffusion of innovations in service organizations: systematic review and recommendations. Milbank Q 82(4):581–629
16. Reason JT (1990) Human error. Cambridge University Press, Cambridge/New York
17. ABIM Foundation. American Board of Internal Medicine, ACP-ASIM Foundation. American College of Physicians-American Society of Internal Medicine, European Federation of Internal Medicine (2002) Medical professionalism in the new millennium: a physician charter. Ann Intern Med 136(3):243–246
18. Smith MA, Bartell JM (2007) The relationship between physician professionalism and health care systems change. In: Handbook of human factors and ergonomics in health care and patient safety. Lawrence Erlbaum Associates, Mahwah
19. Titler MG, Everett LQ (2001) Translating research into practice. Considerations for critical care investigators. Crit Care Nurs Clin North Am 13(4):587–604
20. IOM (Institute of Medicine) (2013) Best care at lower cost: the path to continuously learning health care in America. Washington, DC: The National Academies Press.
21. Casey DE Jr (2013) Why don't physicians (and patients) consistently follow clinical practice guidelines? JAMA Intern Med 173(17):1581–1583

22. Holden RJ, Karsh B (2009) A theoretical model of health information technology usage behaviour with implications for patient safety. Behav Inf Tech 2015/01;28(1):21–38
23. Holden RJ, Carayon P, Gurses AP, Hoonakker P, Hundt AS, Ozok AA et al (2013) SEIPS 2.0: a human factors framework for studying and improving the work of healthcare professionals and patients. Ergonomics 56(11):1669–1686
24. IOM (Institute of Medicine) (2011) Patients charting the course: citizen engagement in the learning health system: workshop summary
25. Pittet D, Boyce JM (2001) Hand hygiene and patient care: pursuing the Semmelweis legacy. Lancet Infect Dis 1(Supplement 1(0)):9–20
26. Gawande A (2007) Better: a surgeon's notes on performance, 1st edn. Metropolitan, New York
27. Grol R, Grimshaw J (2003) From best evidence to best practice: effective implementation of change in patients' care. Lancet 362(9391):1225–1230
28. Best M, Neuhauser D (2004) Ignaz Semmelweis and the birth of infection control. Qual Saf Health Care 13(3):233–234
29. Gurses AP, Ozok AA, Pronovost PJ (2012) Time to accelerate integration of human factors and ergonomics in patient safety. BMJ Qual Saf 21(4):347–351
30. Lankford MG, Zembower TR, Trick WE, Hacek DM, Noskin GA, Peterson LR (2003) Influence of role models and hospital design on hand hygiene of healthcare workers. Emerg Infect Dis 9(2):217–223
31. Shojania KG, Duncan BW, McDonald KM, Wachter RM, Markowitz AJ (2001) Making health care safer: a critical analysis of patient safety practices. Evid Rep Technol Assess (Summ) (43) (43):i–x, 1–668
32. Neuman MD, Bosk CL, Fleisher LA (2014) Learning from mistakes in clinical practice guidelines: the case of perioperative beta-blockade. BMJ Qual Saf 23(11):957–964
33. Shekelle PG, Wachter RM, Pronovost PJ, Schoelles K, McDonald KM, Dy SM, et al (2013) Making health care safer II: an updated critical analysis of the evidence for patient safety practices. Evid Rep Technol Assess (Full Rep) (211)(211):1–945
34. Smith GC, Pell JP (2003) Parachute use to prevent death and major trauma related to gravitational challenge: systematic review of randomised controlled trials. BMJ 327(7429):1459–1461
35. Braithwaite RS (2013) A piece of my mind. EBM's six dangerous words. JAMA 310(20):2149–2150
36. Cabana MD, Rand CS, Powe NR, Wu AW, Wilson MH, Abboud PA et al (1999) Why don't physicians follow clinical practice guidelines? A framework for improvement. JAMA 282(15):1458–1465
37. Lugtenberg M, Zegers-van Schaick JM, Westert GP, Burgers JS (2009) Why don't physicians adhere to guideline recommendations in practice? An analysis of barriers among Dutch general practitioners. Implement Sci 4:54-5908-4-54
38. Weinstein ND (1988) The precaution adoption process. Health Psychol 7(4):355–386
39. Prochaska JO, DiClemente CC (1992) Stages of change in the modification of problem behaviors. Prog Behav Modif 28:183–218
40. Keown OP, Parston G, Patel H, Rennie F, Saoud F, Al Kuwari H et al (2014) Lessons from eight countries on diffusing innovation in health care. Health Aff (Millwood) 33(9):1516–1522

Chapter 8
The Value of Prevention

Matt Mischler and Jessica Hanks

Abstract There is a delicate balance between the cost and the value of health care delivered by medical providers. One specific area in medicine that is continually evolving is preventative care. There are many national organizations who release clinical guidelines on prevention and screening. Clinical guidelines incorporate evidence-based medicine as a means to unify management and minimize practice variation. However there is variability on implementation in clinical practice. The myriad of sources releasing guidelines can create conflict and confusion on the level of the provider and the patient and create difficulty for both in navigating the complex interconnection between cost and value. In Chap. 8, we will focus on breast cancer, prostate cancer, and cervical cancer screening guidelines as examples that highlight this concern. Breast and prostate cancer screening guidelines vary between national bodies and create conflict at the patient-provider level, requiring enhanced communication between provider and patient often without adequate information or knowledge for true informed decision making. Conversely, cervical cancer screening is a success story in screening and prevention given its long-standing history of effectively reducing cervical cancer. It is even more successful in that there is alignment between professional organizations. Finally, we will introduce the concept of medical rationing, which is inherent in the discussion of screening guidelines and their application in clinical practice. For providers, preserving the provider-patient relationship is imperative to the success of any preventative plan and should remain the focus of guideline-driven preventative care.

Past Health-Care Costs

The burgeoning cost of health care in the United States has led to increased attention being paid to the cost effectiveness of numerous medical interventions, including those aimed at preventative care. With the cost of health care at $8,915 per person

M. Mischler, MD • J. Hanks, MD (✉)
Department of Internal Medicine and Pediatrics, University of Illinois College of Medicine at Peoria, Peoria, IL, USA
e-mail: Matthew.J.Mischler@osfhealthcare.org; Jessica.R.Hanks@osfhealthcare.org

© Springer International Publishing Switzerland 2016   97
C. Asche (ed.), *Applying Comparative Effectiveness Data to Medical Decision Making: A Practical Guide*, DOI 10.1007/978-3-319-23329-1_8

in 2012 and with 17.2 % of the economy devoted to health-care spending, the cost of disease prevention is now being measured against the cost of therapeutic intervention [1]. Despite the large segment of the national economy devoted to health care, by many measures the quality of health care in the United States still ranks below that of other industrialized countries [2].

CER is critical to informing which preventive measures should be adopted in health care. Application of CER to specific examples of prevention will be discussed. This topic is worthy because prevention is the key to reducing long- burden of disease and its associated costs.

Preventative health-care measures, including screening tests for primary prevention, have been widely touted as a means of producing cost savings [3, 4]. Studies on the value of prevention and screening, however, have yielded conflicting results regarding cost-effectiveness [3, 5, 6]. Clinical practice guidelines have increasingly been implemented as a means to unify management, minimize practice variation, and standardize practice utilizing the best evidence available to form the basis of the guidelines [7–15]. In order to ensure credibility, well-designed health-care guidelines incorporate evidence-based medicine (EBM) with methods that are transparent regarding conflicts of interest, financial or otherwise, and subjected to a rigorous peer review process [16]. Health-care guidelines that incorporate screening and preventative health-care measures have been issued by large national organizations, as well as by groups of health-care providers who extol expert opinion outside of a national governing body [17].

Despite the increasing use of clinical guidelines throughout all facets of prevention and screening, the impact of these guidelines on clinical practice remains highly variable [18, 19]. With such a proliferation of guidelines arising from numerous organizational bodies, the recommendations and treatment algorithms within the guidelines often provide information that is contradictory or that does not provide clear guidance to the practitioner. Guidelines also require constant updating and refurbishing, with the majority of guidelines showing decreased validity at around 3 years [20]. As a result, medical practitioners are often faced with difficult clinical decisions at the bedside with the patient at the point of care as they struggle to make sense of guidelines that are conflicting and apply the information from the guideline to each individual patient [21, 22]. In addition, barriers to the delivery of evidence-based preventative care are present at all times and must be overcome by the medical provider and the patient alike. Patient-specific barriers such as access to care, and organizational barriers at the local or national level such as inadequate reimbursement and restriction of access, conspire to make the delivery of well-timed, high-quality preventative care difficult [23]. In addition, common themes have emerged that predict medical practitioners' adherence to guidelines, including distrust of the guidelines, conflicting guidelines, interference with the doctor-patient relationship, organizational issues centered around time and reimbursement, and the format and type of guideline provided [24]. These barriers, taken together, inform a larger discussion about not only the quality and utility of preventative care and screening via clinical practice guidelines but also the feasibility at the point of care for guideline implementation by the medical practitioner.

In this chapter, we will outline the common themes of preventative care and screening as they relate to three common diagnoses: breast cancer, prostate cancer, and cervical cancer. These three areas will be highlighted because they currently represent areas of uncertainty and occasional contradiction for providers and patients alike. We will then discuss the impact of rationing care and its impact on guideline adherence. Finally, we will discuss factors that may improve the utility, adherence, and yield of clinical guidelines as they relate to preventative health.

Breast Cancer Screening

Breast cancer is the most frequently diagnosed noncutaneous cancer and the second leading cause of cancer-related mortality in women in the United States [25, 26]. Approximately 1 in 8 women (12 %) will develop invasive breast cancer during her lifetime, with the 10-year risk at ages 40, 50, and 60 being 1.5 %, 2.3 %, and 3.5 %, respectively [27]. Overall, a total of 1 in 36 women (3 %) will die from breast cancer [25]. Given the common occurrence, high level of disease burden, and high mortality rate of the disease, breast cancer often evokes a strong emotional response from a large portion of the medical and lay communities. Therefore, screening for breast cancer also holds a strong spotlight and evokes the same strong response.

As discussed above, professional medical organizations release guidelines for screening tests to provide clinicians guidance in treating their patients. Unfortunately, breast cancer screening guidelines are a high-profile example of duplicity and contradiction in clinical guidelines that can create conflicting pathways for clinicians and patients. In 2009, the United States Preventative Services Task Force (USPSTF) released new breast cancer screening guidelines to great media and public fanfare, with recommendations that limited screening mammography to certain groups and recommended a much more scaled back approach to screening for many women [26]. The result was a swift public backlash from many professional and public interest groups attacking the new guidelines for their limitations in screening [28, 29]. In the creation of the USPSTF guidelines, the task force amplified an already challenging conundrum at the bedside for the clinician, creating guidelines that are discordant with those of the American Congress of Obstetrics and Gynecology (ACOG) and the American Cancer Society (ACS) [30, 31]. This created a rift in guidelines across primary care specialties and made it difficult for clinicians to align their practice recommendations with the guidelines [32].

Following publication of the new guidelines, mammography rates did not decrease across all age groups from 40 to 74 compared to pre-guideline rates, suggesting the guideline did not affect screening rates [33]. With the publication of discordant guidelines, not only were providers potentially confused regarding the correct screening pathway, but a large percentage of women seeking their guidance were as well, with 30 % of women in a recent survey expressing confusion about screening recommendations [34]. The discrepancies among professional guidelines allow a single patient to obtain different recommendations from different providers, creating inherent confusion in the medical system and placing the patient-provider relationship at risk [32].

The heart of the debate over breast cancer screening does not lie in the utility of mammogram as a detection tool for early breast cancer. The initial age at which to begin screening and the interval at which to obtain a mammogram are the major focal points about which the guidelines disagree [34, 35]. The sensitivity and specificity of mammography are reported at 77–95 % and 94–97 %, respectively [26]. The recurring theme in the literature regarding breast cancer screening is weighing the benefits versus the harms of the testing and attempting to define the balance of that ratio over time. The obvious benefit of screening is the potential reduction of breast cancer mortality through early detection. The 2009 USPSTF updated guidelines reported that the number of women needed to invite to screen to prevent one breast cancer death decreased with age. For women 39–49 years old, 1904 women needed to be invited; for women aged 50–59, 1,339 women needed to be invited; for women 60–69 years old, 377 women needed to be invited [26]. The change in the USPSTF guideline recommendations stems mainly from the false-positive rate of mammograms. Currently, 5 % of women with a positive mammogram will end up with a diagnosis of breast cancer after undergoing further testing, compared to 95 % of women with a positive mammogram who undergo additional testing resulting in a false-positive finding [34].

Given the disparity between these major guidelines, how do clinicians assess how to screen, when to screen, and who to screen at each individual bedside encounter? First, the clinician must assess the baseline risk of each patient individually, and this risk must be incorporated into the informed decision-making process about screening. There are statistical models to help estimate each person's risk based on individual patient characteristics. The Gail model and its updated version (Gail model 2) is the basis of the Breast Cancer Risk Assessment Tool through the National Cancer Institute [27]. The model calculates risk based on the patient's medical and reproductive history, prior breast biopsy, and history of breast cancer in first-degree relatives to estimate an individualized risk for each patient. It also has been validated for different ethnicities [36]. Tools such as this can not only help determine risk but can also assess if additional imaging modalities should be used in screening, such as magnetic resonance imaging (MRI). For example, the American Cancer Society recommends MRI if the lifetime risk of breast cancer is >20% [35, 37]. Women with genetic cancer syndromes may benefit from other screening and prevention strategies as compared to the average-risk patient [38]. It is also important to note that for women at higher risk, a negative mammogram may also impart a false sense of security. For example, women with BRCA 1 mutation are at an increased risk of triple-negative breast cancers, which usually are not detected with early screening mammography [39].

In this manner, providing true informed consent for each individual of the risk-benefit ratio of breast cancer screening allows a patient-centered approach for the clinician at the bedside faced with the decision of recommending screening versus non-screening. The benefits of early diagnosis and the effect on mortality, coupled with the harms of false-positive results leading to unnecessary additional workup, overdiagnosis, and psychiatric burden, must be balanced to individualize the decision to screen for each patient [27, 40]. Unfortunately, even with an individualized approach for each patient, there is still wide variation in the expected outcome of the screening process. Estimation of overdiagnosis varies widely in observational studies, from 1 to 10 % to greater than 50 % [26, 27]. The significance of a false-positive mammogram also varies significantly for each woman. While it may increase anxiety and distress regarding mammogram and breast cancer, it does not increase medically diagnosed anxiety or depression [27]. Indeed, false-positive results may increase the rate of breast self-exams performed following the false-positive study [41].

The proliferation of multiple guidelines without clear consensus places the patient and the provider squarely in the middle of the debate when trying to decide the best course of action in the patients' best interest. The strain on the patient-provider relationship due to this divide can have many lasting downstream consequences for adherence in other areas or for trust in the clinician to practice in the patient's best interests. In addition, in the face of contradictory guidance, many practitioners default to defensive medicine, as the guidelines in place to guide decision making unfortunately are perceived to add more risk of litigation [42]. Indeed, some of the main reasons why malpractice claims occur include discounting concerns raised by the family or patient, disregarding and potentially not understanding their perspective, and poor delivery of information from the health-care professional [43]. With discordant guidelines to work from, it is quite easy to see how one, if not all three, of these scenarios can be introduced easily into a patient-provider encounter, increasing the potential for a poor outcome for the patient and the provider.

Given the emotionally charged background of breast cancer screening and the need to maintain the patient-provider relationship, many clinicians base their practice decisions on patient preferences rather than on guideline recommendations [42]. In support of this practice, a cohort of women in the targeted age group for breast cancer screening were surveyed on the 2009 changes to the USPTF recommendations after they read media pieces covering the topic. In total, 86 % did not think the changes were safe, and 84 % of women surveyed were not going to follow them even if it was what their physician recommended. Nearly 50 % of women who thought the new guidelines were safe were still not going to delay onset of screening. Interestingly, women who had had a false-positive test requiring further evaluation in the past did not support the increased interval of screening [44].

As we look at the impact clinical guidelines can have on daily practice and the individual patient encounter, breast cancer is a clear example of the potential for both positive and negative consequences to be introduced into practice through the proliferation of guidelines that are often discordant. The patient and the provider are tasked with discerning the proper path of treatment, with decisions made that may or may not be appropriate or medically sound. However, by taking each encounter individually, a clinician can form a patient-centered approach to the implementation of the guideline and create a "best practice" for each patient encountered with the guideline as a road map. While this does not adhere to the rigidity of each specific guideline, it does allow the plan of care to be tailored to an individual's needs and expectations, something that is vital in the maintenance of the patient-provider relationship and the patient's trust in the provider. Unfortunately, when confronted with the barrier of time required for this approach, organizational barriers limiting clinician decision making, and intrinsic knowledge of each specific nuance of the guideline, the creation of discordant guidelines places unforeseen strain on the provider and the patient, at the peril of the health system.

We will now investigate another conflict in the realm of screening guidelines and preventative care, namely, that of prostate cancer screening.

Prostate Cancer Screening

The appropriate method of screening for prostate cancer, and particularly the role of prostate specific antigen (PSA) in screening, remains extremely controversial. As with breast cancer, there are variation and contradiction in the guidelines issued from different professional societies [45]. Despite varying recommendations to exercise caution in ordering PSA tests, there continues to be an increase in PSA tests performed nationwide [46, 47].

A large part of the challenge in prostate cancer screening is the varying performance of the screening tool, the PSA test. For a PSA level of >4 (need a measurement level for the lab test), the sensitivity and specificity are reported to be 21 and 91 %, respectively, whereas at a threshold level of >3, the sensitivity and specificity are 32 and 85 %, respectively. The level at which to recommend further workup with biopsy is difficult given that up to 9 % of men with PSA <1 had prostate cancer on biopsy [48]. Given the unclear threshold at which a clinician and patient can be confident that disease is not present, and the unclear level at which to initiate biopsy for effective cancer detection, many clinicians do serial screenings of the PSA in follow-up. As a result, an estimated $5.2 million is spent on PSA and any follow-up testing that results in preventing one death from prostate cancer [49]. A recent Cochrane review of five randomized control trials found no significant decrease in prostate cancer-specific mortality with PSA testing, although one study, the European Randomized Study of Screening for Prostate Cancer (ERSPC), found a 21 % reduction in prostate cancer mortality in a subgroup of men aged 55–69 [50]. Comparative effectiveness of alternate screening strategies has shown variation in the degree of decreased mortality, as well as the risk of overdiagnosis based largely on the age at which screening is undertaken [51]. In addition, given the further diagnostic workup required for a false-positive PSA, there is a spectrum of mild to moderate harms associated with screening, ranging from bleeding and anxiety to infection, erectile dysfunction, and incontinence. Abnormal results on a screening PSA may also contribute to overdiagnosis and overtreatment. Again, similar to breast cancer, open dialogue between patients and providers about the balance between the risks and benefits (potentially preventing prostate cancer mortality in approximately 1:1,000 screened men over a decade) is crucial to providing true informed consent and making sense of the conflicting clinical guidelines [52, 53].

Prostate cancer screening is another example of the necessity of shared decision making between a provider and a patient. Shared decision making is defined broadly as two-way exchange of information between the parties concerned with the medical decision at hand, either from the professional or from a patient point of view [54]. When screening guidelines are not clear, the ability of the provider and the patient to engage in shared decision making is crucial to the maintenance of the patient-provider relationship and the delivery of patient-centered care [55].

Recent evidence has shown that several factors affect the rate of screening with PSA, most notably including increasing age and higher levels of education [48]. However, despite the uncertainties surrounding prostate screening, the majority of men report little to no shared decision making with their providers when deciding on PSA screening [56]. If the clinician is unable to engage in shared decision making with the patient, the uncertainty created by inconsistent guidelines will deepen the barrier between the patient and the provider and drive a wedge into the relationship. The clinician must have the toolbox to be able to engage in a shared decision-making conversation with the expertise and communication skills needed to navigate such a high level discussion. There have been multiple reviews regarding how to best develop training for physicians to engage in this discussion regarding prostate cancer screening, with ideas ranging from web-based modules to pre-visit patient education [48, 57, 58]. Unfortunately, multiple barriers similar to those in the breast cancer discussion present the same challenges at the bedside encounter, including time to engage, organizational inconsistencies allowing the clinician to engage, and familiarity and knowledge of the nuances of the guidelines themselves.

With prostate and breast cancer screening providing examples of the challenge clinical guidelines can place at the point of care at the bedside, we will now look at a third example of preventative screening, for cervical cancer, in which there is consistency among national bodies in their recommendations.

Cervical Cancer Screening

Cervical cancer is the third most common cancer in women and the leading cause of cancer mortality in low-income countries around the world [59]. Cervical cancer screening is a "success story" in preventative screening, as the rate of cancer mortality has steadily declined since the introduction of screening [60]. Recently, the USPSTF, the American College of Obstetrics and Gynecology (ACOG), and the American Cancer Society (ACS) revised their recommendations to extend the interval for cervical cancer screening given the known association and timeline of human papilloma virus and cervical cancer [61–63]. The newer screening guidelines take into consideration a woman's age, her personal history, and the type of screening performed. Compared with prostate and breast cancer screening, the main national bodies issuing cervical cancer screening guidelines have uniformity across their recommendations. As with every screening test, the risk-benefit ratio must be evaluated on an individual basis. However, with concordance and clarity in the clinical guidelines, as opposed to contradiction and confusion, this ratio can be discerned more clearly for each individual patient.

Cervical cancer is unique, as it has a known infectious precursor, the human papilloma virus (HPV). This separates cervical cancer from breast and prostate cancer, as it is potentially preventable with appropriate screening. In addition, understanding the infectious timeline and progression from early stage to advanced cancer influences guideline implementation in clinical practice. Infection with HPV results in a range of pathology of varying severity. Most infections are self-limited and cause only transient cellular changes in the cervix [59, 60]. The grade of cellular changes is defined as cervical intraepithelial neoplasia (CIN). The changes caused by HPV range from grade 1 to grade 3. Grade 1 correlates with self-limited infection and regression, not requiring treatment. More frequent cervical cytology examination will detect these self-limited infections and lead to unneeded further procedures. Grades 2–3 involve more cellular inflammation, which requires treatment. If left untreated, the precancer stage of grade 3 will progress to cervical cancer over many years [64]. Given the natural progression over time of HPV infection to precancer and cervical cancer, the minimum age to initiate screening is widely accepted at 21 years, regardless of age at initiation of sexual activity [60–63]. One exception is the CDC's recommendation that HIV+ patients be screened at onset of diagnosis [60].

With a sound understanding of the natural history of the disease, cervical cancer screening guidelines are consistent across all major national organizations with regard to when to begin screening, who to screen, and how often to screen. With consistent guidelines, providers and patients have a strong base to engage in decision making at the point of care.

In addition to clarification of screening interval and population, the type of testing performed for cervical cancer screening has changed as well. With the introduction of HPV screening as part of cervical cancer screening, the sensitivity of the screen for high-grade lesions (CIN 2–3) has increased, while the specificity has slightly decreased compared to cytology of a pap smear alone [65]. As a result of the change in the sensitivity of the screening test, the performance of the clinical guideline must be assessed against the performance of the screening tool. Modeling studies looking at the interval and type of screening done have been performed with the goal of clarifying the proper use of the clinical guideline [66, 67]. In women aged 21–29, it is recommended to do cytology alone every 3 years [61–63]. In other modeling studies, annual screening had slightly better cancer detection rates than screening every 3 years, but there were also significantly more unnecessary interventions performed in women with self-limited infections than when women were screened every 3 years [66, 67]. There was not a difference between screening every 2 or every 3 years [66, 67]. Given that screening yearly versus every 2–3 years resulted in significantly more interventions for positive tests and only a slight benefit in cancer detection, the consensus was to extend the interval to every 3 years in this age group with cytology alone [60]. In women aged 30–65, similar modeling protocols compared results of screening yearly, every 2 years, and every 3 years, with similar results in regard to diagnosis and increased superfluous diagnostic evaluation. Implementation of these guidelines into clinical practice, as supported by the above modeling studies, allows for less overdiagnosis and the avoidance of potential harms due to unneeded workup and treatment. In addition, along with the implications for clinical practice, it has a potential impact on cost-effective medicine and high-value care. Extending the initiation and the interval of screening may reduce both the cost of screening and unneeded diagnostic procedures [60].

The implications of these modeling studies and the resulting impacts on implementation of cervical cancer screening guidelines are profound. In the 1960s, an annual gynecological exam was incorporated into the annual well-woman exam [60]. With the recent changes in the guidelines, there is now a clear indication that such testing is not needed. In stark comparison to breast and prostate cancer screening guidelines, screening for cervical cancer has clearly defined who to screen, how often to screen, and what the resulting benefits are to screening. At the point of care, the ease of use of the clinical guidelines allows for mutual decision making that benefits both the provider and the patient. Since the USPSTF, ACOG, and ACS guidelines are harmonious, cervical cancer screening is streamlined for both the patient and the health-care provider. This creates an environment where the impact of implementation of screening guidelines on cervical cancer rates can be verified and celebrated.

Impact of Variation in Guidelines

As noted through the above discussion, practitioners and patients alike are exposed to clinical practice guidelines for preventative care that often do not create consensus or cohesion among providers. With the difficulty presented to providers in the milieu of preventative care, patients are exposed to similar uncertainty, resulting in wide variation in patient expectations regarding preventative screening. At the heart of preventative screening and clinical practice guidelines is the provider-patient relationship [24]. The implementation of clinical guidelines resulting in successful preventative health care requires stability in the provider-patient relationship, and often, the recommendations brought forward in guidelines involve the rationing of clinical services to what is felt to be the appropriate patient groups [68]. The discussion of not performing preventative services for a patient or patient subgroup, particularly when clinical guidelines are unclear, has the potential to degrade the patient-provider relationship and has led to much debate over the use of limited medical resources [69].

Rationing and Clinical Care Guidelines

Medical rationing is the allocation of scarce health-care resources to those individuals who are believed to derive the most benefit [70]. It is a word that carries strong political and emotional sentiment, particularly in the climate of health-care reform and access to health-care coverage [71]. At the heart of the discussion of preventative care services and the application of clinical guidelines is the idea of the application of services or tests to certain subgroups and the withholding of testing for other groups. Most practitioners acknowledge that some rationing of resources occurs clinically, but there is little agreement on the application of rationing or the proper allocation of resources in the clinical realm [72–74].

When clinical guidelines are created, they inherently create a notion of medical rationing, as some populations are included and others excluded from the focus of a particular guideline. Preventative care and population-based guidelines in general have been raised as an ethical issue unto themselves, with questions of the ethics of screening "healthy" members of the population with testing that has unclear benefit and real risk of harm [75]. As outlined above, there is ongoing struggle with population-based clinical guidelines at the patient-care level, with the practitioner and the patient squarely in the midst of a tumultuous interplay between evidence and real-world application. Patient expectations of screening and of utilization of resources are often at odds with their true requirements according to clinical guidelines, and this can render their impression of the care received as being less adequate [76, 77].

As we see in the discussion above regarding three disease processes for which the medical field recommends screening, the content and consistency in guidelines, which are derived from expert assessment of the evidence, best practices, and expert opinion, directly impact the individual needs of the patient and the provider at each individual encounter. Guidelines often have difficulty finding a common ground and often will place the patient-provider relationship under stress, as the two parties struggle to find a common ground regarding guidelines they may disagree with [78]. In complex decision making that involves the allocation of scarce health-care resources, the physician-provider relationship is the central focus around which decision making is often based. Patients often view their providers as their agents with their best interests at heart, placing trust in the provider to "do the right thing" in each clinical encounter [79]. This implicit trust is the glue that holds the medical system together in the face of often conflicting economic expectations and patient expectations. In a sense, this trust is a substitute for regulations and bureaucracy that may interfere in the patient-provider relationship and is a large factor in decision making in the clinical arena. Competing pressures from patients and professional autonomy, as well as economic factors such as misaligned reimbursement incentives, impact the proper allocation of health-care resources [80]. In addition, patients are often uncomfortable with the idea that their providers must balance the "greater good" with their own good, and they have difficulty making decisions or understanding health care in the context of population-based decision making [81].

As the medical field seeks to improve the utilization of clinical practice guidelines, as well as address the concept of the rationing of scarce health-care resources, it is clear that maintaining the provider-patient relationship is essential to maintaining the integrity, effectiveness, and dissemination of whatever guideline is in question.

Improving the Use of Clinical Guidelines

Within the realm of clinical guidelines and preventative care, for a clinician faced with decision making that impacts an individual patient, numerous factors are involved in the decision to apply a specific guideline or to allocate specific resources toward that patient [24, 68, 69]. For the clinician, the knowledge, attitudes, and behaviors that are exhibited in reference to each patient encounter are highly variable and will often vary from encounter to encounter based on the application of these domains with each individual patient [82]. Targeting these three areas with a consistent point of reference on the provider-patient relationship may hold the key to finding the proper balance between guideline implementation and the allocation of health-care resources.

Knowledge

Clinician knowledge of a specific clinical guideline is influenced by many factors, including familiarity with and awareness of the guideline and its contents. The time needed to stay informed, the clarity of the content within the guideline, and the accessibility of the guideline are large components that inform a clinician's knowledge of a specific guideline [82]. As discussed, guidelines that deal with the same topic but are issued by different bodies often have conflicting content, making it difficult for the clinician to obtain the proper understanding or knowledge of the specific guideline in question [83]. In addition, a practitioner's own experience with a particular subject matter will often inform his or her interest in or ability to obtain knowledge of a clinical guideline [24, 84]. This experience, and knowledge gained through real-world interactions, many times is felt to "trump" the information that is being offered and discussed in a guideline [76, 82, 85].

Overcoming the variability in knowledge of a particular guideline among medical practitioners relies partly on the inherent dedication of the practitioner to ongoing continuing medical education (CME) and remaining current on clinical aspects of care. However, with the time limitations and external pressures placed on medical practitioners in the current health-care system, the acquisition of knowledge and maintenance of specific awareness of guideline content will continue to be challenging. To overcome this barrier, clinicians must be given allotted time away from direct patient care for CME that is focused specifically on guideline familiarity.

Guidelines must be delivered in a useable format that is created considering the practitioner at the bedside who will be delivering the content and executing the allocation of resources. When guidelines on a topic are conflicting, the bodies that have published the guidelines should make every effort to clarify their differences and to provide the practitioner with the rationale behind the differences and the reasons why they differ, with some consensus reached that is applicable to the real world. In doing so, the guideline must remain "user friendly" and must be applicable at the bedside in order for a patient-provider encounter to remain meaningful and productive. Finally, maintenance of guidelines within the electronic medical record (EMR) domain may help to improve knowledge centered on a specific clinical guideline. With the incorporation of the EMR across inpatient and outpatient domains, interfacing with the EMR in a streamlined fashion with helpful clinical decision guides may assist clinicians in maintaining knowledge of a particular guideline as it is applicable to each patient encounter. The decision aids, however, must allow flexibility for each individual patient, as very few patient encounters will entail the identical interface with the guideline in question.

Attitudes

The attitude of a practitioner toward a guideline, and thus toward allocation of resources, is a major determining factor in the likelihood of a practitioner to utilize the guideline [24, 82, 84]. Skepticism toward the validity of a particular guideline, particularly when the guideline is conflicting with another or has a hint or potential of bias, will influence the likelihood that clinicians will implement the guideline at the bedside [86, 87]. Conflicting attitudes toward the practitioner's role in the rationing of health-care resources is a large component of variability in the application of clinical guidelines [88]. The concept of the practitioner as a "double agent" has been discussed to describe the conflict between provider testing and prescribing patterns and the administrative monitoring of health-care expenditures by individuals without direct ties to patient care [89]. The possibility that a guideline may interfere with the patient-provider relationship also exerts a large influence over the attitude of a provider toward a particular guideline and its implementation [83].

To improve the attitude of a practitioner toward a particular guideline, the guideline itself must first prove to be patient centered. With the patient-provider relationship at the heart of the discussion at the bedside, a provider must know that the guideline in question will allow him or her to deliver patient-centered care focused on the well-being of the individual he or she is caring for. Skepticism, particularly when guidelines conflict, needs to be cleared through comparative effectiveness trials and systematic reviews that can establish the superiority of a practice or test over another and provide a "real-world" recommendation to the practitioner that is applicable. With transparency and integrity infused into a guideline, and with the goal at the heart of the guideline clearly being the well-being of the patient, the attitude toward a particular guideline will be much different than that toward a guideline that lacks a patient-centered focus. Guidelines that are distanced from the patient, or that attempt to place the provider at a distance from the patient, will be looked upon negatively and will be poorly adhered to. Providing a clear understanding in the particular guideline of the impact at a patient-specific level, and acknowledging variations in practice due to individual patient factors, will allow a guideline to be more patient centered and patient specific and thus looked upon more favorably.

Behaviors

The behavior of a clinician in the delivery of care is affected by many factors, including knowledge and attitudes that inform the decision-making process [24, 82]. Often, factors that exert pressure upon the practitioner, either internal or external to a specific organization, will exert influence within a patient encounter [90]. The inability to reconcile patient preference with a clinical guideline, the perceived threat to the integrity of the patient-provider relationship, and even the length of the relationship itself will affect the behavior of a clinician in the clinical arena [83].

To improve the behavior of a provider with a particular guideline, the goals and incentives at organizational level, be it hospital, practice, or payer, must be aligned to reinforce the best outcome for the patient. When goals are misaligned and unclear, a provider will lose faith in a particular guideline, and adherence to that guideline will be lost. The methods that are incentivized must be patient centered, and they must be clearly tied to the guideline to reinforce the patient-specific outcome in question. There must be flexibility within the guideline or organizational structure itself to allow a clinician the ability to make adjustments for each individual patient, and there must be an allowance for individualizing the plan of care when it is in the best interest of the patient as deemed necessary by the clinician. The clinician must be allowed to act as the patient advocate in a way that advances the best outcome for the patient, preserves the patient-provider relationship, and allows the clinician to act as a steward of resources in a rational, patient-centered manner [91].

Conclusion

The application of clinical guidelines to patient care has the potential to standardize care, reduce health-care waste, and provide a road map for clinicians to better care for their patients. However, features inherent in common guidelines raise challenges for clinicians and patients and affect the utility of and implementation of many commonly used clinical guidelines. At the heart of each clinical guideline are the patient-provider relationship and the need to maintain the integrity of that relationship for both the patient and the provider. With the need to allocate scarce health-care resources adequately now greater than ever, the clinician must be given the tools to engage in a meaningful dialogue with his or her patients while maintaining the trust inherent in the relationship. It is through this relationship that we will carry health care forward and move into a more sustainable and equitable model of care, with clinical guidelines as the road map for both the clinician and the patient. If the patient-provider relationship is fractured or lost, no guideline in existence can repair that relationship.

References

1. Chokshi DA et al (2012) The cost-effectiveness of environmental approaches to disease prevention. N Engl J Med 367(4):295–297
2. Davis, K et al (2014) Mirror mirror on the wall, 2014 update: how the U.S. Healthcare System Compares Internationally. The Commonwealth Fund. http://www.commonwealthfund.org/publications/fund-reports/2014/jun/mirror-mirror#. Published: 16 June 2014. Accessed: 28 Sept 2014
3. Cohen JT et al (2008) Does preventive care save money? Health economics and the presidential candidates. N Engl J Med 358(7):661–663
4. Hengstler P et al (2002) Evidence for prevention and screening: recommendations in adults. Swiss Med Wkly 132(27-28):363–373
5. Krogsboll LT et al (2012) General health checks in adults for reducing morbidity and mortality from disease. Cochrane Database Syst Rev 10:CD009009. doi:10.1002/14651858.CD009009.pub2
6. Boulware LE et al (2007) Systematic review: the value of the periodic health evaluation. Ann Intern Med 146(4):289–300
7. Vaughn TE et al (2002) Organizational predictors of adherence to ambulatory care screening guidelines. Med Care 40(12):1172–1185
8. Fang E et al (1996) Use of clinical practice guidelines in managed care physician groups. Arch Fam Med 5(9):528–531
9. Solberg LI et al (2000) Lessons from experienced guideline implementers: attend to many factors and use multiple strategies. Jt Comm J Qual Improv 26(4):171–188
10. Pearson KC (1998) Role of evidence-based medicine and clinical practice guidelines in treatment decisions. Clin Ther 20(Suppl C):C80–C85
11. Davis DA et al (1997) Translating guidelines into practice. A systematic review of theoretic concepts, practical experience and research evidence in the adoption of clinical practice guidelines. CMAJ 157(4):408–416
12. Mittman BS et al (1992) Implementing clinical practice guidelines: social influence strategies and practitioner behavior change. QRB Qual Rev Bull 18(12):413–422
13. Woolf SH (1993) Practice guidelines: a new reality in medicine. III. Impact on patient care. Arch Intern Med 153(23):2646–2655
14. Woolf SH et al (1999) Clinical guidelines: potential benefits, limitations, and harms of clinical guidelines. BMJ 318(7182):527–530
15. Weisz G et al (2007) The emergence of clinical practice guidelines. Milbank Q 85(4):691–727
16. Raine R et al (2005) Developing clinical guidelines: a challenge to current methods. BMJ 331(7517):631–633
17. DeMaria AN (2006) Populism in guideline writing. J Am Coll Cardiol 48(5):1109–1110
18. Grimshaw JM et al (2004) Effectiveness and efficiency of guideline dissemination and implementation strategies. Health Technol Assess 8(6):iii–iv, 1-72
19. Lomas J et al (1989) Do practice guidelines guide practice? The effect of a consensus statement on the practice of physicians. N Engl J Med 321(19):1306–1311
20. Shekelle PG et al (2001) Validity of the Agency for Healthcare Research and Quality clinical practice guidelines: how quickly do guidelines become outdated? JAMA 286(12):1461–1467

21. Lawrence MR (2001) Give us clear, not convoluted, clinical practice guidelines. CMAJ 165(11):1468
22. Niederhuber JE (2002) Seeking calmer waters in a sea of controversy. Oncologist 7(3):172–173
23. Rubin HR (2000) Overcoming barriers to preventive care. J Gen Intern Med 15(6):434–436
24. Carlsen B et al (2007) Thou shalt versus thou shalt not: a meta-synthesis of GPs' attitudes to clinical practice guidelines. Br J Gen Pract 57(545):971–978
25. What are the key statistics about breast cancer? Am Cancer Soc. http://www.cancer.org/cancer/breastcancer/detailedguide/breast-cancer-key-statistics. Revised: 25 Sept 2014. Accessed: 20 Oct 2014
26. Nelson HD et al (2009) Screening for breast cancer: an update for the U.S. Preventive Services Task Force. Ann Intern Med 151(10):727–737, W237-42
27. Pace LE et al (2014) A systematic assessment of benefits and risks to guide breast cancer screening decisions. JAMA 311(13):1327–1335
28. Mitka M (2013) Physicians, patients not following advice from USPSTF on mammography screening. JAMA 309(20):2084
29. When evidence collides with anecdote, politics, and emotion: breast cancer screening (2010) Ann Intern Med 152(8):531-532
30. American College of Obstetrics and Gynecologists (2011) Practice bulletin no. 122: breast cancer screening. Obstet Gynecol 118(2 Pt 1):372–382
31. Can breast cancer be prevented? Am Cancer Soc. http://www.cancer.org/cancer/breastcancer/detailedguide/breast-cancer-prevention. Revised: 25 Sept 2014. Accessed: 22 Nov 2014
32. Corbelli J et al (2014) Physician adherence to U.S. Preventive Services Task Force mammography guidelines. Womens Health Issues 24(3):e313–e319
33. Pace LE et al (2013) Trends in mammography screening rates after publication of the 2009 US Preventive Services Task Force recommendations. Cancer 119(14):2518–2523
34. Breast cancer: when and how often to get screened. How do you make sense of conflicting mammography guidelines? (2013) Harv Womens Health Watch 21(2):3
35. Can breast cancer be found early? Am Cancer Soc. http://www.cancer.org/cancer/breastcancer/detailedguide/breast-cancer-detection. Revised: 25 Sept 2014. Accessed: 21 Oct 2014
36. Breast cancer risk assessment tool. Natl Cancer Inst. http://www.cancer.gov/bcrisktool/Default.aspx. Accessed: 25 Oct 2014
37. Graubard BI (2010) Five-year and lifetime risk of breast cancer among U.S. subpopulations: implications for magnetic resonance imaging screening. Cancer Epidemiol Biomarkers Prev 19(10):2430–2436
38. Marmot MG (2013) Breast cancer screening recommendations—reply. JAMA 310(19):2102
39. Lannin DR (2014) Risk and benefits of screening mammography. JAMA 312(6):649
40. Miller AB et al (2014) Twenty five year follow-up for breast cancer incidence and mortality of the Canadian National Breast Screening Study: randomised screening trial. BMJ 348:g366
41. Brewer NT et al (2007) Systematic review: the long-term effects of false-positive mammograms. Ann Intern Med 146(7):502–510
42. Meissner HI et al (2011) Breast cancer screening beliefs, recommendations and practices: primary care physicians in the United States. Cancer 117(14):3101–3111
43. Beckman HB et al (1994) The doctor-patient relationship and malpractice. Lessons from plaintiff depositions. Arch Intern Med 154(12):1365–1370
44. Davidson AS et al (2011) Attitudes of women in their forties toward the 2009 USPSTF mammogram guidelines: a randomized trial on the effects of media exposure. Am J Obstet Gynecol 205(1):30.e1–7
45. Mitka M (2013) Group now advises against routine PSA screening. JAMA 309(22):2316
46. Virginia A. Moyer (2012) on behalf of the U.S. Preventive Services Task Force (2012) Screening for Prostate Cancer: U.S. Preventive Services Task Force Recommendation Statement. Ann Intern Med 157(2):120–134
47. Hamoen EH et al (2013) Discrepancies between guidelines and clinical practice regarding prostate-specific antigen testing. Fam Pract 30(6):648–654

48. Hoffman RM (2011) Clinical practice. Screening for prostate cancer. N Engl J Med 365(21):2013–2019
49. Brett AS et al (2011) Prostate-cancer screening—what the U.S. Preventive Services Task Force left out. N Engl J Med 365(21):1949–1951
50. Ilic D et al (2013) Screening for prostate cancer. Cochrane Database Syst Rev 1:CD004720
51. Gulati R et al (2013) Comparative effectiveness of alternative prostate-specific antigen—based prostate cancer screening strategies: model estimates of potential benefits and harms. Ann Intern Med 158(3):145–153
52. Dahm P et al (2013) Screening for prostate cancer: shaping the debate on benefits and harms. Cochrane Database Syst Rev 9:ED000067
53. McCarthy M (2013) Evidence does not support routine PSA testing, say experts. BMJ 346:f2982
54. Charles C et al (1997) Shared decision-making in the medical encounter: what does it mean? (or it takes at least two to tango). Soc Sci Med 44(5):681–692
55. Kasper J et al (2012) Turning signals into meaning—'shared decision making' meets communication theory. Health Expect 15(1):3–11
56. Han PK et al (2013) National evidence on the use of shared decision making in prostate-specific antigen screening. Ann Fam Med 11(4):306–314
57. Wilkes M et al (2013) Discussing uncertainty and risk in primary care: recommendations of a multi-disciplinary panel regarding communication around prostate cancer screening. J Gen Intern Med 28(11):1410–1419
58. Feng B et al (2013) Physician communication regarding prostate cancer screening: analysis of unannounced standardized patient visits. Ann Fam Med 11(4):315–323
59. Wheeler CM (2013) The natural history of cervical human papillomavirus infections and cervical cancer: gaps in knowledge and future horizons. Obstet Gynecol Clin North Am 40(2):165–176
60. Karjane N et al (2013) New cervical cancer screening guidelines, again. Obstet Gynecol Clin North Am 40(2):211–223
61. Moyer VA et al (2012) Screening for cervical cancer: U.S. Preventive Services Task Force recommendation statement. Ann Intern Med 156(12):880–891, W312
62. Committee on Practice Bulletins – Gynecology (2012) ACOG practice bulletin number 131: screening for cervical cancer. Obstet Gynecol 120(5):1222–1238
63. Saslow D et al (2012) American Cancer Society, American Society for Colposcopy and Cervical Pathology, and American Society for Clinical Pathology screening guidelines for the prevention and early detection of cervical cancer. Am J Clin Pathol 137(4):516–542
64. Hariri S et al (2011) Prevalence of genital human papillomavirus among females in the United States, the National Health And Nutrition Examination Survey, 2003–2006. J Infect Dis 204(4):566–573
65. Arbyn M (2006) Chapter 9: clinical applications of HPV testing: a summary of meta-analyses. Vaccine 24(Suppl 3):S3/78–89
66. Kulasingam SL et al (2013) Screening for cervical cancer: a modeling study for the US Preventive Services Task Force. J Low Genit Tract Dis 17(2):193–202
67. Stout NK et al (2008) Trade-offs in cervical cancer prevention: balancing benefits and risks. Arch Intern Med 168(17):1881–1889
68. Mechanic D (1997) Muddling through elegantly: finding the proper balance in rationing. Health Aff (Millwood) 16(5):83–92
69. Bradley CP (1992) Factors which influence the decision whether or not to prescribe: the dilemma facing general practitioners. Br J Gen Pract 42(364):454–458
70. Scheunemann LP (2011) The ethics and reality of rationing in medicine. Chest 140(6):1625–1632
71. Bloche MG (2012) Beyond the "R word"? Medicine's new frugality. N Engl J Med 366(21):1951–1953
72. Hurst SA et al (2006) Prevalence and determinants of physician bedside rationing: data from Europe. J Gen Intern Med 21(11):1138–1143

73. Strech D et al (2009) Are physicians willing to ration health care? Conflicting findings in a systematic review of survey research. Health Policy 90(2-3):113–124

74. Ward NS et al (2008) Perceptions of cost constraints, resource limitations, and rationing in United States intensive care units: results of a national survey. Crit Care Med 36(2):471–476

75. Skrabanek P (1990) Why is preventive medicine exempted from ethical constraints? J Med Ethics 16(4):187–190

76. Peck BM et al (2004) Do unmet expectations for specific tests, referrals, and new medications reduce patients' satisfaction? J Gen Intern Med 19(11):1080–1087

77. Zemencuk JK et al (1998) Patients' desires and expectations for medical care in primary care clinics. J Gen Intern Med 13(4):273–276

78. Beaulieu MD et al (1999) Practice guidelines for clinical prevention: do patients, physicians and experts share common ground? CMAJ 161(5):519–523

79. Mechanic D (1995) Dilemmas in rationing health care services: the case for implicit rationing. BMJ 310(6995):1655–1659

80. Carlsen B et al (2005) "Saying no is no easy matter" a qualitative study of competing concerns in rationing decisions in general practice. BMC Health Serv Res 5:70

81. Mechanic D et al (1990) Choosing among health insurance options: a study of new employees. Inquiry 27(1):14–23

82. Cabana MD et al (1999) Why don't physicians follow clinical practice guidelines? A framework for improvement. JAMA 282(15):1458–1465

83. Tudiver F et al (2001) Making decisions about cancer screening when the guidelines are unclear or conflicting. J Fam Pract 50(8):682–687

84. Langley C et al (1998) Use of guidelines in primary care—practitioners' perspectives. Fam Pract 15(2):105–111

85. Worrall G et al (1996) Hope or experience? Clinical practice guidelines in family practice. J Fam Pract 42(4):353–356

86. Zyzanski SJ et al (1994) Family physicians' disagreements with the US Preventive Services Task Force recommendations. J Fam Pract 39(2):140–147

87. Siriwardena AN (1995) Clinical guidelines in primary care: a survey of general practitioners' attitudes and behaviour. Br J Gen Pract 45(401):643–647

88. Cooke M (2010) Cost consciousness in patient care—what is medical education's responsibility? N Engl J Med 362(14):1253–1255

89. Shortell SM (1998) Physicians as double agents: maintaining trust in an era of multiple accountabilities. JAMA 280(12):1102–1108

90. Vaughn TE et al (2002) Organizational predictors of adherence to ambulatory care screening guidelines. Med Care 40(12):1172–1185

91. Pearson SD (2000) Caring and cost: the challenge for physician advocacy. Ann Intern Med 133(2):148–153